Vaporizing Medical Marijuana: Volume
420
(Omicron vaporizer v2 plus Hexane
Honey Oil-Bonus: Vol. III #1 BestSeller,
Vol. II, "Vaporizing Medical Marijuana #1
BestSeller" & grow Medical Marijuana
guide, butter recipe, make concentrates
& Hashetone)

By Dr. Jacob Ray

Prologue-

The rapidly evolving world of technology surrounding the pen vaporizer revolution has prompted another volume in this series. Thank you and welcome to the fun and comprehensive Volume 420! I have included all three previous volumes to illustrate how quickly they become outdated after being on the shelf for less than six months. Volumes One and Three have become bestselling ebooks in that time. I wanted to fan the flames by adding a fourth volume to update readers on the latest Omicron v2 and include tips for crafting hexane honey oil. The previous volumes feature plenty of basic information about the Vapir bag inflatable, the Vapir NO2, the Magic Flight Launch Box, the Arizer Solo, and the Omicron pen vaporizer. The cartridges and tips included in volume three for the Omicron are compatible with the new version or v2. The guidance around crafting your own concentrates is worth keeping. I will add more tips for readers who are looking for new semi solids to load or dab. This volume will focus on the everchanging

Omicron pen vaporizer as it is the only one that offers refillable cartridges. I will also impart some new findings around cartridge weights before, during, and after use. This volume is an amalgamation of countless hours spent researching various devices and methods of crafting concentrates. San Francisco is the birthplace of medical marijuana and will remain our example for comparing other tolerant cities. The market for concentrates in San Francisco has exploded. Many dispensaries are carrying several top shelp waxes, budders, and oils. The prices range from $35-60 a gram depending on the solvent used and method of extraction. If you are located in a state with tolerant laws but limited concentrates, this volume will guide you in crafting your own. In the quest for purity of process, I have researched more on vacuum purging and discovered an affordable alternative for patients who only need to craft small batches of concentrate for their safe consumption. My philosophy is to provide patients with the basics and allow them to refine their process through preference plus trial and error.

Use what works. Use what strains you find medicinal or therapeutic. But, consider your long term health if you are still combusting your medical marijuana. Convection promises longevity. Combustion equals massive carcinogen intake from the burning of leafy material alone. If you cannot part with the flame, try vaporizing anyway. You might enjoy the flavor profiles. Give those tired lungs a break and hop on board. I promise you a safe journey. If you still have questions after reading all four volumes in this series, get online. Reach out to the medicating consumers. We are a family. And, we are here to help. Forums can provide information, promote unity, and foster fellowship. Find a thread that speaks to you and tell them I sent you. I keep this series free for Prime folks and ninety-nine cents to everybody else to provide you with the basics about vaporizing medical marijuana. Pay it forward by joining the medicating consumer community. You are never alone. And, curiosity begets education. We need each other to advance this movement towards compassion. I hope you will do your part to celebrate and lift up the joy of this ancient healer our country foolishly banned so long ago. Unbind yourselves from the laws of man and let nature heal you with cannabis. Let it give the sick an appetite so they can eat. Let it halt the nausea brought on by Wasting Syndrome. Let it calm the storm of anguish in the mind of the depressed patient. Let it take away the aches and pains from the gravity of this world. Beneath our foolish laws lies a teacher and a prophet. She comes to us from antiquity to heal modern woes. We cannot silence her as she is nature. She is more pure than this corrupt man made world can conceive. Her voice is a whisper or a thunder. It rings out through the valleys of despair. It drains the water around the island of pain and shows you the path to glory and health. We, as men, can no longer hold her back. We must nurse from her bountiful bosom and rejoice at her power to heal. We must turn to her and stop running away. If you are politically torn but a medicating consumer, I urge you to pledge allegiance to her, your healer. She gave you what you did not or could not have had otherwise. Time to return the blessing. Vote to keep medical marijuana pure and accessible. It is time to rise up and be heard together.

Chapter 1- How fast technology changes around vaporizers and how to shop with that in mind.

If you haven't bought a vaporizer, chances are you are open to suggestion around what your medicating needs require versus which type of vaporizer is right for you. If you are madly in love with flowers (buds) but are hesitant around concentrates due to chemicals or processes used to make them, know that your fears are justifiable. There are plenty of examples of bad concentrates. But, there are ways to identify a bad concentrate and we will go over those in more detail later.

Before deciding on a vaporizer, you should answer the following questions:

How much money do I have to spend?
Do I want portability?
Should I consider a home unit and a portable?
Based on my tastes and preferences, do I want flavor or extraction of THC/CBD only?

If I purchase a vaporizer, can I reliably acquire or craft my own concentrates to use?

Knowing that I can use vaporized medical marijauna in edibles, how much money will I save on my medical marijuana purchases if I vaporize instead of combust? Do I require medicating daily? If so, should I switch to vaping to reduce carcinogens? What if things change and my clubs close, can I acquire medical marijuana or concentrates from growers or private caregivers? What does the local law say about how much medical marijuana I can have in my possession? Would using a vaporizer help reduce the amount of medicine I need to carry or conceal? Can I handle the increase in potency that comes with using concentrates? Am I prone to panic attacks, paranoia, or increased anxiety when medicating with potent medical marijuana? If so, is vaping a better alternative due to dose regulation? Do I want a vaporizer that has to be plugged in to work? Should I purchase an additional charger for travel or to have on hand?

How much time do I have to research the existing market for product and price comparisons on vaporizers? Should I buy a used vaporizer?

The great news about this series is I have done tons of research and field tested several dependable, affordable vaporizers for you. I wrote all of these volumes with the medicating consumer on a budget in mind. The vaporizers detailed and compared in the series retail for just over a hundred, with the exception of the Arizer Solo which retails for closer to one fifty. If you have money for medical marijuana, chances are you have some reserved for your current methods of getting medicated. That is, if you are rolling joints, you buy papers and lighters. But, you are bombarding your system with smoke, which might lead to cancer or other respiratory problems, like Chronic Obstructive Pulmonary Disorder. Why chance it? Vaporizing is as clean as It gets while providing the illusion of smoke. The flavor produced from vaporizing is far superior to any combustion method. Once vaporizing takes hold of your medicating experience, you will no

longer enjoy combustion. Like the
former cigarette smoker who sneaks a
drag years later and coughs, you will
taste the heat from combustion,
carcinogens, and burned leafy matter.
Dabber purists might disagree with me.
Some medicating consumers will say
they love their smoke. I am open to
being enlightened but I will put my
Omicron up against any other flavor out
there. Once you find or craft top shelf
wax, budder, oil or CO2 extract and
draw from an Omicron, you will rejoice
at the instant relief and flavor. Potency is
a flavor in its own right. That is not
unique to medicating with concentrated
marijuana. If I compare beers, I would
say drinking cider is like vaping flowers
whereas drinking barleywine is like
vaping concentrates. The flavor is more
robust and hearty. It is an acquired
taste. Vaping flowers is as delicious as
drinking cider or a light beer but vaping
concentrates is comparable to adding
the potency factors into flavor. A
barleywine with twelve percent alcohol
paired with a hearty flavor to reflect that
strength becomes more potent by
design just as the well crafted
concentrate boasting seventy percent

THC does. Potency, flavor, effect, and method of use combine to envoke the need for a vaporizer in your life. Try it. You might be shocked at the brand new way to enjoy your favorite strain's full flavor profile and healing power. Some medicating consumers will spend a fortune on medical marijuana only to discover the combustion based methods they use are toxic or that they are vaporizing many of the psychoactive components before they can be absorbed from the temperature of the heat source being too high. If you hold a lighter flame onto a burning bowl of medical marijuana, you are inhaling post-combustion butane by product and smoke. You are also burning off THC and other psychoactive cannabinoids. Heat vaporizes THC. That's why you don't use your microwave to dry out fresh clipped buds. Heat from any source can vaporize THC. That is why all of the old school whip based vaporizers and other borderline combustion based and butane powered vaporizers were discluded from these volumes. Too much heat is too much heat. Too much unregulated heat is even worse. The Omicron meters and regulates doses and heat. The Arizer Solo features some heat regulation. It has heating increments from one to seven. You should vape flowers on the two setting and finish them off by increasing the temperature to three then four. Never go over four, the Arizer gets too hot. The Vapir bag inflatable and NO2 feature temperature controls. Try vaping hash at 350 degrees through your Vapir bag inflatable after fluffing it and filling the bowl a third of the way. It works but any more heat would make it too hot to inhale without coughing. Which leads me succinctly to another test of heat index: coughing fits. If you have inhaled medical marijuana that was too hot, chances are once it got into your lungs it expanded and caused you to cough. Coughing can be unpleasent and painful. It can sometimes get scary. Patients who are weak from their ailments want to reduce coughing fits. Those who have atrophy as part of their spectrum of symptoms will want to reduce coughing fits as they can exhaust the diaphragm.

If you are still not convinced that vaporizing is the way to go for health and flavor, let's conduct an experiment.

You will need the following items to see the difference in combustion and convection using a Gravity bong:

1. A pitcher (with a handle) large enough to accomodate a large clear plastic soda bottle
2. Two emptied large clear plastic soda bottles. The bigger the better.
3. Scissors and clear packing tape.
4. A glass bong bowl piece (not the female stem inserted in the bong, the bowl piece)
5. A lighter
6. A small knife or paper clip or safety pin
7. A water source
8. Concentrate or semi solids

Instructions:

Step one- Cut the bottoms off of the emptied clear large plastic soda bottles. Only cut off the bottom inch. You want as much of the bottle as possible. Keep the caps they came with.

Step two- Heat the knife with the lighter and carve a hole in the top of one of the caps big enough to accomodate the glass bowl piece from your bong. Use the clear packing tape to seal around it. Get an airtight seal. You will not be pulling the glass piece out so make sure its secure and airtight. On the other emptied bottle with the bottom cut off, heat the knife and carve a hole big enough to accomodate the Omicron detachable mouthpiece that affixes to the end of the cartridge. Make sure the hole is positioned so that the Omicron remains horizontal or angled slightly down. Use the clear packing tape to secure the mouthpiece and creat an airtight seal. Fill the pitcher with water leaving an inch or two of space from the top. Take the caps off of both emptied soda bottles. One has the glass piece, the other is unchanged.

Step three- Start by placing the glass piece modified bottle into the pitcher filled with water. Allow it to sink to the bottom completely. Load your concentrate after screwing the cap on airtight. Using the lighter, catch the concentrate on fire as you are slowly pulling the bottle up creating a vacuum with the water. The bottle will fill with smoke. Unscrew the glass piece modifed cap. Hold the bottle in place and seal it with your mouth. Allow the bottle to sink and push the smoke into your lungs as you inhale. Be careful not to do this too fast as you will spill water everywhere. You can put a ping pong ball into the water between the bottle and pitcher to stop water from gushing out in the combustion set up. Repeat the process until you are medicated. Allow the medication to cycle through.

Step four- Remove the glass piece modified bottle. Place the Omicron modified bottle into the pitcher filled with water. Now, place your Omicron onto the sealed mouthpiece located on the side near the top of the emptied soda bottle with the bottom inch cut off. Press the button as you lift up creating a vacuum. The bottle will begin to fill with vapor. Even if you have the v2 Omicron, do not hold the button down the whole time. Toggle on and off in increments of eight to ten seconds or you will overtax your battery. A stream of vapor should appear. Tease it up slowly until it fills the bottle completely before inhaling it in by removing the Omicron then the cap and sinking it while inhaling. Repeat until medicated.

Step five- Continue alternating between bottles for at least a week. After substantial use, remove both bottles for comparison. Notice how much cleaner the Omicron bottle is when compared to the other. Smell them both. The Omicron smells sweet. The amount of visible build up found in the combustion based gravity bong should convince you of how carcinogenic or tarry combustion can be, even when using concentrates. This test should be replicated using all glass and rubber seals. I am confident any researcher would agree the proof lies in the residue left behind: none for the Omicron and dense coating for the glass piece combustion set up. Try it for yourself. This experiment should sway even the staunch skeptics. Be sure to compare the experiences of medicating from either set up. Most users report a cleaner, longer lasting, better quality buzz from the vape set up. The flavors from set up to set up are markedly different. The combustion smoke can be harsh and cause coughing fits whereas the Omicron vapor cloud produced in the vacuum can be as large but have no expansion from overheating. The resulting cloud is smooth, visible, but purely vapor and surely contains less tar and carcinogenic toxins. Only a well funded lab can prove me right or wrong but if you want to see what your lungs look like from combusting, take a look at the bottle after a few months of heavy use. The Omicron set up is still crystal clear due to no build up. The sides of the combustion set up are opague with tarry residue and build up. Use clear plastic bottles (not colored ones) to best see the outcome. You can also use the bottle to meter or consolidate dosing. The gravity bong does all the work. Let it. All you have to do is lean over and inhale. Keep in mind that the gravity bong packs a solid punch when using flowers and concentrates. Be prepared to cough and pay the price if you test the limits it can go. The smallest effective dose should be the golden rule but most medicating consumers enjoy medicating and the rituals that come with it. Have fun medicating but eliminate or at least reduce carcinogens with a vaporizer. The other reason I selected the Omicron v2 for this volume is a cartridge is in development for flowers and concentrates. Those cartridges will be reloadable. Therefore, the Omicron is a sound investment for the $129.00 range as it will soon be able to vape anything.

For medicating consumers who want all glass when vaping or the closest thing to it, buy the Arizer Solo. It can vape flowers and hash. You need to fluff out your hash before loading it. You can craft a third bottle for the gravity bong set up to add to your experiment with vaping versus combusting at home. Be careful when detaching the Arizer from the bottle after pulling it up as the glass whip mouthpiece slides out easily. If you vape hash using the Arizer do not heat past two or three or you will cough. Use dense hash.

Any hash or semi solid that liquifies will not work in the Arizer without flowers to act as medium for it. Sandwich the liquifying types between a top and bottom layer of flowers. Otherwise they will liquify and could clog the airholes inside the ceramic chamber that houses the glass mouthpiece. The Arizer should never be held from the bottom as there are airholes there as well. Flip it over and inspect it with the mouthpiece out. Cover the bottom forming a seal with your palm and dry hit it. The Arizer Solo features a new straight, four hole mouthpiece. This is ideal for added airflow when compared with the curved, two hole mouthpiece that it comes with. The straight piece cleans with ease. Please refer to the first three volumes for more tips and information about the Arizer. I have had mine for almost a year and it works great. It wastes no medicine. All medicine you run through it can be retained and used in making medicated butter. Refer to volume one for the recipe. The Arizer paired with the Omicron can meet and exceed your need for vaping flowers and concentrates. Buy 'em all. You will rediscover them over and over while reducing your risk-benefit ratio for respiratory disease when comparing to combustion. And don't worry skeptics, the relief is evident in proper use of the vaporizers compared here. I have combed the forums. I have read all the reviews for you. I assure you the vapor movement is your friend. Let's save a life: yours. Tell your patient friends or ask to try one of their vapes. Be sure to

read the return policies for vaporizers.
Use common sense by not shipping any
vape back with medical marijuana
residue on it. Many vendors know
people won't risk jail to ship it back.
They claim they can't issue a refund
without the vape itself. Check before
you buy if you buy online. If you buy
from a store or club, check the return
and refund policy. Some stores will not
take a vape that has been used for
medicating. They will state that it was
sold for legal not illegal use. Even in
tolerant states, stores will refuse
returned merchandise with residue or
any use that is questionable. Be careful
of bargains and bundles of vapes with
other merchandise. Gifts are great but
don't hesitate to find out about the
warranty on the vape. Be leery of
websites outside your country of origin.
If something goes wrong, you definitely
shouldn't risk sending it back if it has
been used. Drug dogs can smell any
amount of residue. Shop for any other
vapes at your own risk. I can only vouch
for the ones I have field tested: the
Omicron, (first generation, described in
volume three), the Arizer Solo Portable,
the Vapir bag inflatable, the Vapir NO2

Portable, the Magic Flight Launch Box and the latest Omicron v2 (Version Two). The changing technology has reached a plateau with the advent of the Omicron and its refillable cartridges. Vape developers will focus on glass components and battery life. But, until a vape comes out that is ready at the push of a button with extremely potent concentrate from a refillable glass cartridge, I'm sticking with the Omicron. Don't spend too much money on any vape. Next year or in two years another one will come out that vapes better. Save up for that day. The vapes discussed here fall short when compared to the latest Omicron but they are still a blast to have around. This journey has been scary, especially when I thought the tumor I had might be malignant but this amazing plant has kept me writing and positive. These incredible, revolutionary medical devices have provided the vehicle to salvation. The least I can do is tell you how to get there using them safely while you are in need.

Chapter 2- A detailed description of the Omicron v2, the latest pen vape by THC Scientific

The latest Omicron pen vape features several innovative changes. The biggest change is the addition of removable, rechargeable batteries that load from the unscrewed bottom. The battery is placed and the bottom screws in and lights the LED light on the button. Cartridges screw in and now feature the derlin mouthpiece. Users can lock their Omicron by following the instructions in the User manual included in the kit for safe pocket transport. The carrying case is sleek and houses all components securely and with style. The kit includes a refill tool and empty cartridge. The charger for the batteries features a collapsable plug for easy transport. Be careful when plugging the charger in. Place the battery(s) before plugging in. The folding plug will slip sometimes and free itself from the plug while you are trying to insert the battery. The spring loaded metal piece on the charger that slides to house the battery for charging should be handled carefully as it snaps with a surprising amount of force. Don't touch the metal contact points while its plugged in. The carrying case does not house the charger. The charger does not feature a USB charge option like the original Omicron did. The Omicron v2 contact point found at the center and bottom where the cartridge screws in must also be wiped down with isopropyl alcohol between uses due to the occasional leaky cartridge. The contact point is slightly different for the Omicron v2 in that it has a recessed trough across the middle. The Omicron v2 battery hugs the cartridge. This new closeness is slightly different than the original Omicron which has deeper ridges which could impact airflow. The Omicron v2 is a little taller than the original. It does not include an optional outer metal sleeve like the original did. The Omicron v2 button can be pressed and held without autoshutoff kicking in after six seconds. Users should not hold the button continuously as this rapidly depletes batteries, cartridges, and concentrate. Try releasing the button after ten seconds for larger hits. If you want massive vapor hits buy the Persei by THC Scientific. They also make the Omicron and the Persei fits one or two cartridges for patients who want bigger vapor hits. The Persei retails for two hundred. It has an attachment called the Hammer for dabbers. There's another vape called the O-PHOS which appears to be a plug in or portable Omicron that charges from the bottom via USB. The flower and concentrate cartridge is coming soon. Visit them online at delta9vapes.com for more information.

The original Omicron featured a charger that attached to the contact point. This was changed due to chargers getting sticky and shorting out or breaking from leaky cartridges. Who is to blame? Bad concentrates. Top shelf concentrates almost never leak. The charger works fine if it is wiped down between uses with isopropyl alcohol. Mine has lasted for months. You can also wipe the bottoms of messy cartridges. You can scrub the threadings and should periodically do so. Always use isopropyl alcohol to wipe down components. Cartridges that are placed around dusty areas pick up dust. Wipe everything down before and after use to preserve your investment and maximize efficiency of use. Cartridges weigh 7.8 grams empty and 8.6 grams loaded with one gram. Buy some digital scales and monitor how much you have left in your cartridges and shop accordingly. The Omicron v2 comes in two colors. The outside is sleek and has no rough edges. The draw from it seems somewhat reduced compared to the original Omicron but the concentrate used also factored in. Good concentrate vaped great in both Omicrons. Some stubborn experimental cartridges and other heavy use cartridges vaped better or produced a thicker stream on the gravity bong set up described above when attached to the original Omicron. The Omicron v2 battery seemed a little less powerful when fully charged unless I was vaping expensive top shelf wax or oil. The theme here is that what you vape with impacts the Omicron's overall performance. This leads to a brief discussion of spotting bad concentrates.

Bad concentrates:

1. Smell like the solvent used to craft them. That is, if you go to sniff some Butane honey oil or budder or wax and it stinks of butane, pass on that

batch. Clean extractions should minimize the solvent's presence as much as possible. Smell is an important test that should be done before you buy. If they won't let you smell it before buying, be leery. Ask how it was made, who made it from what, and exactly which solvent was used. If you get a batch that smells bad as soon as you put heat to it, get your money back.

2. Bubble up or expand when heated. When cheap butane is used (or other diluted solvents) the final product tends to bubble up. It might look great until you try to get it loaded into your cartridge. You begin priming it and might even get a few draws before it bubbles up and over the sides of the cartridge and onto everything else. If you smell butane or hear bubbling, stop heating it. You may have a dirty or cheaply made concentrate.

3. Are black or dark brown when made with alcohol. Pure isopropyl alcohol or pure grain alcohol is used to extract oils. The problem is alcohol also breaks down chlorophyll which effects the color and taste of the oil.

The Omicron cartridges are not made for alcohol based oil extracts. Be sure to ask if alcohol was used to make the concentrate before loading it for use with the Omicron.

4. Come at bargain prices. If a gram of oil or wax or budder is on sale or cheap, it was made poorly most of the time. You get what you pay for. Clubs have set the price of top shelf concentrates to reflect the price of eighths of flower. A gram of semisolid supposedly equates to 4.5 grams of flowers. But, that says nothing about potency. Well crafted concentrates are sometimes seventy to ninety percent THC. Go ahead and shop around but usually a twenty-five dollar gram smokes like a twenty-five dollar gram. That thirty-five dollar gram isn't as good as the fifty-dollar one but its way better than the cheap stuff. If you can't afford the good stuff, make it yourself.

The medical marijuana you purchase, grow, refine or change should be consistently clean and as pure as the wind driven snow. The better quality or sparkly potent buds they sell you at the overpriced profit driven nonprofit dispensary might seem worth it but make sure they test it. Make sure the concentrates you buy liquify with heat before loading them for use with the Omicron. Never try to load hash. If you craft your own concentrates be sure to refine them all the way. If you are in the market for reliable clubs or dispensaries read reviews on Yelp and weedmaps.com. Always ask if tax is included in the price before purchasing anything from a dispensary or club. If you are looking for specific concentrates or strains, check forums and search local websites from clubs and dispensaries. Some clubs record their menu in a daily message. Shop around and compare strains and types. Competing dispensaries must offer specials to retain patient members. Some offer coupons on weedmaps.com. San Francisco delivery dispensaries offer a free gram of anything on the menu with your fifth order or ten percent off of concentrates when you order before noon, or they bundle flowers with concentrates by offering honey oil buds. Dispensaries that hoard their meds and jack up the prices under the guise of compassion give the medical marijuana movement an obstacle to overcome together: greed. We can help weed these places out (pun intended) by refusing to spend money there. If you are surrounded by clubs and dispensaries that are all overpriced (common in southern California) spend extra time shopping around. Specials and online coupons offer a fun way to look for bargains and save money. Remember: Isopropyl or alcohol hash oil (usually dark green or black from too much chlorophyll) is not optimal for the Omicron. Make sure the hash oil you purchase is made using isomesmerization. Ask employees and managers. If they duck and dodge or tell you it will work, use an older cartridge. Older cartridges are great for prototype homecrafted concentrates from your private stash or for testing the low end club's taffy or wax. New cartridges should be reserved for master crafted medicine. Order a box of five cartridges for variety. Building a tolerance is inevitable when you buy tons of the same concentrate. Keep a variety to maintain relief. Some patients will enjoy keeping several strains for various uses and times of the day. For example, a patient may start their day with a Sativa like Trainwreck wax and after dinner they might medicate with an Indica like a Grandaddy Purple hash oil. They might add a third or fourth varietal the next day to stave off tolerance building and to maintain symptom relief. Solvents used in making medicine for the Omicron can vary greatly in quality, purity, and byproducts produced but at least you are vaping it and not catching it on fire. The risk-benefit ratio is so greatly reduced by using convection not combustion it confounds the claim that marijuana can cause cancer. Vaping reduces toxins but by how much? We don't know. But, it is visibly evident when you examine the corroded glass pipe of a heavy medical marijuana smoker and the mouthpiece from a heavily used Omicron. Smoke leads to ash. Vaping leads to vapor and when using flowers, edibles. Which one is more cost effective? Which one is better for the human race? Which one would you give to a dying friend? I would hand them the Omicron. Until there's a vape that is ready at the push of a button with high percentage THC concentrate through all glass reloadable parts, I'm sticking with the Omicron. The metal cartridges are durable and hardly impact flavor. But, my imagination drifts to a glass reloadable cartridge of the future capable of vaping even the tiniest amount of anything.

Chapter 3- Hexane Honey Oil & other concentrate tips, vacuum purging update.

Hexane is another solvent that can be used to craft a loadable semisolid concentrate for use in the Omicron. Be sure to shop around for reagent grade hexane in its purest form (99.8%). There is a product for cleaning contacts with hexane and a propellant, some patients use it. I would only trust the purest hexane. If you are making a batch for your Omicron, you will need shake or sugarleaf trim, at least. I will focus on the process and let you determine how much you are willing to attempt. Start small. I won't detail how to do large batches for that reason. Hexane and all solvents used to make concentrates are to be respected. Avoid all flame sources, pilot lights, or burning red embers. Some patients fear having a lighter in their pocket or their cell phone. You be the judge. Be overly cautious. Hold off on medicating until after you craft concentrates. Foolish mistakes can ruin a batch and delay your being able to medicate further. Stay focused and alert for changes in the viscosity and fumes from heat being applied to a concentrate. If your finished product smells or tastes anything like gasoline, you need to refine it further and not consume it until it has no residual smell from the hexane.

You will need the following items to craft Hexane Honey Oil/Wax/Budder:

1. Hexane
2. A new glass Mason jar
3. Unbleached coffee filters that fit over the unopened jar
4. Shake or sugarleaf trim (at least an ounce) ground up fine but not powder fine
5. A medium size pyrex dish
6. A large pyrex dish that accomodates the medium dish with room to spare for water
7. A heat plate
8. Razors or metal scraping tools
9. Water
10. Kettle

Step one- Make sure the shake or trim is ground up but not to powder. Fill your Mason jar with the shake or trim. Go outside away from any and all flame sources. Pour hexane over it. Cover all the shake or trim. Allow the hexane thirty minutes to work. Place it in a dark or shaded area if possible. While it soaks outside, boil water.

Step two- After thirty minutes, place the large pyrex dish down and then the medium dish inside of it. Fill with boiling water and float the medium dish. Pour the hexane extract from the jar through a coffee filter into the medium dish. Allow all of the liquid to pass through the filter. Discard the soaked trim and shake. Set the empty jar aside.

Step three- Continue to swap out the boiling water as the hexane evaporates off. If your hexane won't budge, add water to it enough to float it and continue to add boiling water beneath it in the large dish. The extract will accumulate around the dish. Scrape it off. Once all of the water and hexane has evaporated (you will know by smelling it for any gasoline-like aroma) scrape it off.

Step four- The next step involves taking the scraped up hexane honey oil/wax/

budder and spreading it and whipping it while it sits in another fresh pyrex dish on the heat plate or griddle. Too much heat will evaporate the THC. Keep the temperature low. Continue to whip the extract until it takes on a semisolid state at room temperature. Smell it as it is purging. Smell the final product before using. If you smell any gas-like smell, keep whipping and heating. If you cannot rid the final product of residual smell or any suspect qualities, don't risk medicating with it. The final extract (if adequately purged) should liquify with heat and load easily into an Omicron cartridge. For bigger batches, use a bigger jar, more hexane, and be prepared to battle to get it all evaporated. Heat purging will work as long as temperatures are kept low enough to avoid vaporizing the THC you have worked so diligently to obtain.

Some patients may wish to spends a few hours online reading forums and watching youtube videos on crafting concentrates to refine their approach or learn what not to do. Reading, asking questions, watching videos, and consulting manuals like this series is a great foundation. But, don't neglect your health. Spend as much time as you need researching before you dabble with crafting. The outcomes can range from anger to bliss. Knowledge and troubleshooting will come from researching this fun way to get medicated. Don't skimp on the details.

Speaking of details, I wanted to update my tip section and instructions for vacuum purging butane honey oil by suggesting an affordable product called the Vacu Vin Coffee Saver Starter Kit. Once you blow your butane and heat purge, (read the previous volumes for more details on making butane honey oil) place it inside the Vacu Vin. The Vacu Vin features a hand pump that removes air from the chamber. Remove the air from the chamber and allow the butane honey oil to bubble up. After a few minutes, release the valve allowing the butane honey oil to bubble back down. Repeat this purging process at least five times or until there is little to no bubbling. You can also heat the butane honey oil using the water bath method between vacuum purges. The Vacu Vin is ideal for small batches.

When crafting small batches of butane honey oil, try a glass turkey baster with the ball detached. Flip it over and fit it with an unbleached coffee filter over the wide end after stuffing it with shake. Blast your butane through the narrow end and into your pyrex dish. There are glass butane extraction tubes online for forty grams but for smaller batches, try a glass baster. Don't grind your shake or trim into powder for making any concentrate. Remove all sticks, stems, and other coarse plant matter. Dark final products mean too much chlorophyll was absorbed. The taste or flavor could be compromised. Try soaking for less time if your concentrates are coming out dark or taste bad or bland.

Keep it safe. Keep it clean. Have fun. Be careful. Research everything before your first atttempt. When medicating, think of those people who put their lives on the line or who sit in a Jail cell for breaking the law to push the agenda this world must come to accept as truth: marijuana is medicine. If euphoria, laughter, an appetite, and better sleep are side effects and we can now vape and avoid carcinogen overdosing, let's pledge to stamp out the flames from combustion. Use butane to make butane honey oil for vaping instead of using it to combust flowers and concentrates. The future of vaping starts with you.

Dedication: to Karma delivery & Waterfall Wellness in San Francisco. Keep up the great work! To the Stanley brothers of Colorado, keep up the fight! We are rootin' for ya!

Coming soon: Volume Five & Advocating for the Medicating Consumer

Thanks to all my readers, the global readership is incredible and life giving! I love you all! Thanks for feeding my family & letting me guide you towards healthy medicating!

Vaporizing Medical Marijuana III:

"It looks to me to be benign."

The relief washed over me as Dr. Mickel let me know the good news. Last year, my speaking voice had become raspy. I had a sore throat that lingered. I read up on various cancers before concluding that my past addiction to cigarettes had come back to haunt me in the worst way. I was convinced I had laryngeal cancer from all the carcinogens I had inhaled. Thankfully, my love of music was to blame. I had a benign granuloma on my right vocal cord positioned on the cord itself. I knew carcinogens could not be part of my using medical marijuana to treat my condition. They had caused me to panic enough. I looked to vaporizers for relief. Edibles were also a fun way to medicate but the lipids used to make them coupled with my sweet tooth made them too fatty and easy to build a tolerance to by the end of the batch. I yearned for smoke. I hated saying goodbye to the rolling papers, blunts, glass pipes, one hitters, and all my combustion powered medicating devices. But, they had to go. I shed a tear as I gave each one a new home to my fellow patient friends. I bought the

Vapir bag inflatable. It showed up fast. I fell in love with bag vapes. I had used the Volcano but it was so far outside my budget. It remained unobtainable. I loved the sessions using the Vapir. They were great for medicating groups of patients. The books included below talk about the Vapir in detail and how to use it. If you love flowers, grab one. The next party you throw with other patients, take the other piece of hose that comes with it and blast the whole group. The idea is to huddle around and pass it as it kicks out flower vape from the tube. Have all three containers packed and ready. Patients will love the nonstop stream of dense vapor it produces. The other vaporizers I bought and tested are included below in the two prior volumes on vaporizing with medical marijuana. They include: the Magic Flight Launch Box, The Vapir NO2 Portable, & the Arizer Solo Portable vaporizer. If you like vaping flowers, read up on which device best fits your needs and budget. If you are ready to enter the future of medicating, I invite you to consider the Omicron. Volume three on vaporizing medical marijuana will focus exclusively on the Omicron pen vaporizer and the concentrates used in its reloadable cartridges. There are dozens of pen vaporizers ('pen' here means magic marker, sharpee, or ink pen-sized devices) on the market. The Omicron has been selected for several reasons. The two most important being the reloadable cartridge feature and warranty on the battery. For those of you who are new to pen vaporizers, they are basically comprised of a battery and a screw on cartridge. Some have a third component called an atomizer which screws in between battery and cartridge. The cartridges have one end to attach to the battery and the other end is where the vapor comes out upon inhaling either through an attached mouthpiece or capped end. There may be many other features and designs available. This volume will focus on the Omicron due to the extensive field testing I have put it through. I will discuss the world and market for concentrates used in the Omicron. I will use the San Francisco dispensary market as an example of how concentrates are changing the medicating consumer. But, most of all, I will educate you on what you are investing in with the Omicron versus any other pen vape on the market. I have researched many pen vapes. But, I keep reaching the same conclusion: why bother with any pen vape that doesn't feature reloadable cartridges and a year warranty on the battery? Plus, I have been using the Omicron for three months. Is it perfect? No. Do cartridges clog? Sometimes. Do I lose product from the bottom? Rarely, but it happens. Does having to wipe the terminal with isopropyl alcohol before each charge get annoying? Yes. Have I had to buy a new charger due to a minor design flaw? Yes. So, why am I so amped to share this amazing device? Because it works and if anything goes wrong, I call the sales rep for San Francisco (who is also a patient) and he comes to my home to replace it. Living in this city has an obvious advantage. For those of you reading who have problems with your device, I implore you to not ship it back if it might have gotten medicine on it. Even trace amounts of THC are easily sniffed out by drug dogs. Don't chance it. Don't buy your Omicron from websites based outside of the United States. It will take forever to get to your house. I got duped on my purchase from a

Canadian website. They promised free shipping. The Omicron took forever to get here. It was tracked but sat in Customs for days. Get it from the same website you got this ebook. If they are out of stock, check back. Buying from the manufacturer is fine but the fees stack up. There's a significant handling fee, for example. I made the mistake of hanging my Omicron from the charger which caused the delicate wiring inside to come apart at the contact points. The manufacturer updated the user manual included in all kits to prevent charger problems. They also added the recommendation to wipe down where the charger screws in with isopropyl alcohol before each charge. Even a tiny amount of leakage from the cartridge bottom is enough to interfere with the connection over time. And, some concentrates will leak. Poor quality ones are prone to leak the most. The best news came from the Canada website (once I informed them my unit was malfunctioning) when they had the local sales rep contact me about a replacement. The next day, they showed up with a full replacement, including a new charger. This is great news for me but for those of you in states who are new to the medical cannabis movement, this will be a dealbreaker. Before you decide against purchasing an Omicron because I damaged mine but happened to be in a city with a sales rep, consider all vaporizers bought online. If you're using it to medicate you are taking a huge risk in shipping it back if something goes wrong. Vendors won't refund your credit card without the faulty device. So, any purchase made online is a gamble regardless of return policy. The Omicron is a workhorse. The perfect union of device and concentrate has culminated with the advent of Pure Gold hash oil by Tetralabs. The future of medicating has arrived. Let's medicate together using this amazing device paired with this incredible concentrate. If you live in California, you are set. For my readers in other states, I invite you to take a glimpse at the future. California is the home of Pure Gold and the Omicron. Since I am spending a fortune to live here, I will be your guide. The Omicron can be purchased online. But, what are you going to do about concentrates? Don't worry. If you have access to medicine, you can craft your own concentrates. They might be rough around the edges but they will do. I have included the previous volumes in this ongoing series below. There are some guidelines for researching how to craft concentrates for use in your Omicron. The only addition in this volume to the list of concentrates that will work in your Omicron is hashetone. Here's how you make it: first, purchase 100% pure Acetone with no additives. Do not use finger nail polish remover with scents, additives, or any thing like that. You want beauty salon grade Acetone. You want the bottle to say "100% Acetone." Any other type of Acetone might have chemicals that will coagulate on your lungs. You need a small, sanitized or brand new glass jar. Make sure the lining on the bottom of the lid is not plastic. Plastic may leech into your solution as you are performing a quick wash. You will need to fluff four grams of hashish and place it in the jar. Make sure the hashish is broken down to its smallest size. Get a timer. Set it for three minutes. Pour enough acetone to cover the hashish by an inch. Put the lid on tight. Start the timer. Begin <u>vigorously</u> shaking the jar. Take an unbleached coffee filter and carefully pour the solution through it and into a medium size Pyrex bowl. Have a larger bowl with hot water in it to float the Pyrex bowl as the solution is poured in. The heat from the hot (not boiling, just hot) water will aid in the evaporation of the acetone. Swap the water out once it gets warm. Let all the acetone evaporate and dry. Hover over the bowl sniffing for acetone. Do you smell acetone? Then, it isn't ready. Remove the remaining semi solid from hot water. Allow it to dry. Take two brand new razors and scrape the semi solid off the Pyrex. Spread it back out. Scrape it up again. You will continue to scrape and spread the hashetone until you get a firm semi solid. You should spend an hour spreading and scraping. Smell the semi solid. Does it smell like Acetone? If so, keep spreading, scraping, and sniffing until it smells like hash. Take your empty Omicron cartridge. Hold it from the bottom. Insert the refilling tool. Before loading the hashetone, apply heat to both the cartridge and filling tool while holding the bottom. Do not heat where the threads are. Use your fingers to gauge heat index. Too hot to touch means you might be vaping the THC or melting seals inside the cartridge. Scrape the hashetone into the filling tool. Melt it into the cartridge making sure to continually heat the length of the cartridge to make sure the hashetone slides down into the chamber. Don't heat the bottom. Stop heating the last quarter of the cartridge. The hashetone will bubble up and protest going into the cartridge but slowly heat it and let it make its way inside the chamber. You will want to allow the cartridge to cool for fifteen solid minutes before attempting to vape. The most important thing to keep in mind is to coax the vapor out using a sipping motion. Draw the vapor in <u>slowly</u> to your oral cavity. Then, take it into your lungs. There is no need to hold it in. But, continue drawing air through the cartridge after your hit to cool it off and retain airflow through the airtube. If your hashetone came out more solid than liquid, you may have some clogging. Do not use guitar strings to poke cartridges. Most are made from metal alloys that turn brittle after too much heat. That causes them to snap. You can ruin a cartridge by having a piece of metal shear off inside it while trying to unclog.

If you do have to poke a cartridge, go slow. Angry jabs and frustrated stabs ruin cartridges and limit access to the product inside. If you cannot draw air through your hashetone, make the next batch thinner by using more acetone to make it more liquid. Crafting semi solids is an art. Using solvents can be toxic or fatal. Acetone is extremely flammable. Don't make hashetone indoors. And, stay far away from any open flame source. Tell smokers to stay away or do it when they aren't around. You shouldn't risk blowing yourself up over crafting concentrates. If you are afraid, don't dabble in crafting. Leave it to the pros or move to California and get it from Tetralabs. Hashetone tends to evaporate from cartridges and should be capped when not in use. Hashetone will vary per extraction method used in the hash you made it with. If you are hesitant to try hashetone, go for budder which is butane honey oil that has been whipped while in the same hot water bath until it resembles butter. Butane honey oil should be made with the most refined butane you can find. It should also undergo vacuum purging. There are many methods to sucking the air out of a container with your batch of honey oil on a piece of parchment paper. The idea is to remove all impurities. Purging can and should be repeated several times. Hashetone is less labor intensive but many patients fear using acetone. As with all solvents, there are variables such as how they were made using what and the risks of ingesting harmful chemicals leftover from extracting. With vacuum purged extracts, the proof lies in the final product. Well purged butane honey oil is superior to hashetone and costs much less to produce. Shop around for which method of vacuum purging fits your budget, if you attempt to make butane honey oil or budder. There are glass extraction tubes available online for making butane honey oil. Many extractor tubes are made of plastic or PVC pipe. Stay away from plastic when crafting, storing, or handling semi solids. There is a chance the plastic could leech into your semi solid. Don't use plastic syringes to fill your Omicron cartridges with heated concentrates. Glass is better and can be heated to extract all of your concentrate. Using plastic syringes wastes product as you cannot apply heat to get it to liquify to pour out once it has had time to cool off. When heating a glass vial or syringe, heat the length of the container first to liquify the semi solid trapped inside. Do not overheat. You will vaporize the THC. Heat the glass to expedite the flow of the semi solid out of the container and into your cartridge. Use vicegrips or clamps if you need to steady the cartridge during filling. If you are clamped in, be sure to keep applying heat to the cartridge and filling tool. Otherwise, the semi solid won't make it into the chamber. You will have problems using it and might get angry. You need to keep the cartridge heated but not overheated. Semi solids entering an overheated metal cartridge will vaporize the THC. Be careful. Stay away from the bottom with the lighter and if you use a torch lighter, be extra careful. Some users suggest keeping your torch on the lowest setting and keeping the tip of the flame close but never touching the cartridge while moving It quickly to make sure heat is evenly distributed and only sufficient to get the liquified semi solid moving into a hot enough cartridge. If you purchase a semi solid and it comes in a plastic container (common in San Francisco) make the same hot (but not boiling) water bath. Float the container in the water bath. Some containers are tiny and require dunking. Don't dunk them underwater. Keep the water at the brim while submerging the container for several minutes. It should liquify. I suggest using a glass syringe to get it out and into your cartridge. There will be some product stuck inside the glass after you squeeze it out. Apply heat to get it all. There will be some char build up on the outside of the glass syringe from heating but it wipes right off. Some dispensaries carry Canna Nectar in gram size doses in a plastic syringe. Those are ideal for the Omicron as the gram of nectar is liquified as it is pushed out by the plunger. Press the syringe opening alongside one of the cartridge side slots after preheating your cartridge. Plug the airtube in the middle with the tip of a toothpick if you want to avoid getting any semi solid on or in the airtube. Squeeze the nectar into the slot and apply heat to the whole top three-quarters of the cartridge to help it reach the chamber. Heat the top one third of the cartridge anytime you see any

amount of semi solid collected there.
The cartridges can handle some abuse.
But, they perform better when stored
upright at all times. Never allow full
cartridges or your Omicron with the
cartridge attached to lie on its side.
Even when transporting the Omicron
don't allow it to get sideways in your
pocket. Find a heavy, tall enough, roomy
enough cylinder-shaped bowl to store
cartridges upright. Keep your eye on the
threaded end of the cartridges as they
tend to pick up debris. If you get a leaky
cartridge, store it in a container that can
be heated so you can reclaim lost
product. Another important cartridge tip
is that overheated semi solid coupled
with overheated cartridge causes
leakage from the bottom. I bought a
$35.00 wax from my local dispensary. I
had no problem grabbing the glob of
wax out and stuffing it into the filling tool.
I had preheated and began heating the
wax to liquify it into the cartridge. It took
a long time to liquify a full gram while
applying heat to the cartridge top three-
quarters and filling tool. The heat from
the wax caused it to expand and bubble.
Once it entered the overheated cartridge
it had no where to go as the increased

heat caused further expansion and the result was wax coming out of the bottom. I had coincidentally placed the cartridge on a tile surface and was able to scrape the wax, smear it alongside the slot opening and melting it back into the cartridge but there was a significant amount of wax lost on the threading which had to be wiped clean with isopropyl alcohol to prevent it from collecting on the charger and battery. Once that cartridge was going, it tended to experience the same problem with leakage with repeated hits. That same cartridge is still in use and when loaded with well made hash oil, it functions fine. This horror story brings me to the crux of my argument: buy the Omicron and use Pure Gold hash oil.

Let's put on our thinking caps and explore the world of concentrates, how they are made and from what, and how some clubs are making a fortune off of medicating consumers new to the vape pen revolution by selling overpriced one time use cartridges for other pen vapes.

Part 1- The wide world of medical marijuana concentrates.

Anything from hashish to kief, wax to CO_2 extract, or budder to liquid tincture is considered a concentrated form of marijuana. The Omicron can handle all semi solids. And, soon will be able to handle hash and flowers. The Omicron developers are working on a cartridge for flower and hash enthusiasts. It should be out by March, 2012. There is a video on youtube showing the inventor of the Omicron testing it out with obvious success. The website delta9vapes.com has this cartridge in the catalog with "coming soon" in the product description. The Omicron can use virtually any preloaded cartridge, if you purchase the adapter set. I have used the adapter(s) to field test other cartridges and they work great. This makes almost any cartridge you find usable. The problem with most preloaded cartridges is twofold. The first trap is the one time use feature. Clubs want you to keep paying them too much for cartridges. Most of them wave the banner of being compassionate and nonprofit based. This is bullshit. They are just as slimy as the Republicans trying to shut them down. They are all about profit margins. Don't be fooled by clubs promising their cartridges are the best, most potent. It is impossible to beat being able to fill your own cartridges with any semi solid you'd like. Clubs in San Francisco overprice preloaded cartridges and fly the banner of compassion to get you on board. They carry some type of vape pen that only takes their cartridge. Then, they lock you in to buying your preloaded cartridges from them. One club boasts a whopping twenty-five dollar preloaded glycerine bound cartridge. This is still a ripoff. Glycerine bound preloaded cartridges promise lofty THC levels when in fact, they cannot compare to vaping pure hash oil or Pure Gold hash oil. Glycerine bound THC cartridges are a rip off, across the board. Stay away from the clubs who offer a vape pen and their own preloaded cartridges. You will waste money and tax your lungs trying to catch half the buzz you would from real hash oil without glycerine. The preloaded cartridges have a cotton filament inside saturated in glycerine bound THC solution. The end of the cartridge tastes terrible as the cotton and plastic components succumb to the heat. Some clubs use a tincture bound with glycerine. They claim the THC levels to be comparable to the tincture which is chemically impossible. Glycerine limits how much THC can bind. If you need more proof, buy an Omicron and adapter set. Go to a club with preloaded cartridges. Buy one. Make sure it fits one of your adapters and vape it using your Omicron. Have another cartridge of a quality semi solid that you loaded. Compare and contrast. The buzz from the pure cartridge will win everytime. Glycerine bound cartridges might taste great. They might get you a solid head change. But, they simply cannot compare to pure semi solid cartridges. And, if they are good, what are you going to do once that club goes out of business or continues to jack their price up? Clubs know medicating consumers are drawn to novelty and potency. But, any club offering preloaded cartridges, even with great semi solids, is ripping you off. Load your own cartridges. That way, you see and inspect what is going into your body. You know it is pure, uncut concentrate and that you are getting the most bang for your buck. There are some clubs that carry preloaded Omicron cartridges. I can't imagine a low enough price to make them worth purchasing. Always ask clubs if their prices include tax. Tax on semi solids can raise the price so much it makes more sense to shop around. Go to weedmaps.com and research your local dispensaries. Notice how many offer preloaded cartridges and a pen vape for one to two hundred dollars. If they carry Omicron cartridges, consider that no matter how you slice it, you are getting burned on price. How do I figure? Let's take a quintessential ripoff club based in San Francisco. They feature dozens of strains and plenty of great concentrates. They even sell the Omicron and a few varietals of preloaded Omicron cartridges. The Omicron cartridges retail for $70.00 plus tax! This is a total ripoff as one could purchase a five pack of Omicron cartridges online for fifty dollars, making each empty cartridge only ten dollars. You could shop around for semi solids and buy a gram from $35-50 and load that saving at least ten dollars or much more. You could possibly craft a gram of butane honey oil and drive the price down even further. The Omicron challenges the user to shop around. Once you accept that club prices are set to make profits for nonprofits and will go nowhere but up as the popularity of pen vapes spreads, you will start to revisit crafting your own semi solids. I suggest spending hours on youtube researching various methods to making semi solids before picking the method that fits your comfort and skill level. Be sure to respect the materials you will be handling. Flammable means make it outdoors. If you are nervous, shop around for the best price on semi solids and bypass the make-it-yourself route. If you decide to make your own, research it thoroughly. This guide is meant to give you a framework but you are expected to take the reigns when it comes to your medicine. I am not liable in any way for anything that you do after reading this or any of my books. Use caution and common sense. If you make a semi solid and are hesitant to try it for any reason, listen to that voice. Cut your losses. Keep your body healthy. Concentrates used in vaping come in many forms: hashish, kief, butane honey oil, hexane oil, alcohol based hash oil (does not work well in Omicron), earwax or wax, budder, glass, shatter, hash oil, tincture, CO_2 extract, hashetone, and glycerine bound tinctures used in cotton filament cartridges. Clubs that don't test their products for THC content and impurities are to be avoided. I suggest calling clubs and asking two questions before joining. Do they test everything on their shelf? And, do they charge tax or is it included in the total price? Again, clubs will try to claim that their top shelf stuff is the best, that first time members get a few gifts, and that their meds are all organic. If they don't use lab testing, you never know what you're paying for. Growers for clubs are into quantity and adequate quality. Strains that are robust and resilient, trendy and potent are chosen over weaker, less popular strains prone to problems. Growers work to have the fastest turnaround on the best product. What makes you think using any chemicals that work to meet that goal isn't standard operating procedure? Growers use anything that works once bugs or mold infest crops to try to salvage what they can from it. Clubs that don't test strains and all products they sell for consumption are in cahoots with shady growers. Afterall, they are both making a fortune while the medicating consumer thinks they are getting a bargain. If you have been wondering why I have pushed for Pure Gold hash oil (over all other concentrates) is they test their products. They use isomesmerization to craft superior oil and it shows in the taste and quality of vapor produced. The combination of a reloadable cartridge and lab tested pure hash oil trumps all other pen vapes and preloaded concentrate filled cartridges on the market. The only forseeable downside to using only Pure Gold is building a tolerance to it. My prediction is that Pure Gold per capsule comes from a variety of plants and might stave off tolerance building but not for heavy medicators. That is why it can be fun to experiment, shop around, and find other semi solids you can enjoy between Pure Gold refills. Save a cartridge for experimental semi solids if you are making your own. The only real guarantee to getting pure product is to grow it yourself. This takes at least five months. While waiting for your crop to finish, shop around for semi solids.

Part 2- How to be an informed
medicating consumer

Here are some questions to ask or
consider when buying from clubs and
vaping:
1. After researching this club online
   before going, by reading all the Yelp
   and Weedmaps reviews, and any
   other resource where medicating
   consumers discuss the place, do I
   like what I hear and see?
2. Is my current club adequate for my
   needs? Should I venture out if my
   favorite club has what I need, even if
   the price is higher?
3. Do I want my medicating experience
   to be based on getting meds from a
   place where I can also socialize or
   see the same faces?
4. Do I want a community based club or
   a clearinghouse with bargains?
5. Should I consider delivery based
   clubs?
6. How will I get to the club? Is that
   method of transport reliable?
7. How important is my private
   information's (such as my
   photocopied Identification and
   recommendation) safety? Should I

ask the club or dispensary how and where my personal data is stored? And, if they give out my information if the club is closed or investigated by local, state, or federal authorities? Could I be arrested for belonging to a club which operates outside the law even if I am unaware of them doing so?

8. Should I consider producing my own medicine? If so, should I find a club that sells clones or start with seeds? How much money could I save by growing? If I opt to grow will my power company notice a spike in my power bill once my lights are turned on? Could I be reported to the authorities for producing a spike? Are medical marijuana patients in my area allowed to grow? How much? Where can I read the local laws before growing in order to be compliant?

9. Does the price I see on the club menu include tax? Is tax worth paying if it drives the price up higher than other clubs that include tax?

10. Does this club's medicine work?

11. Is a one time gift worth joining a club whose prices are too high?

12. When buying concentrates for the Omicron, should I go for variety, strength, novelty, or consistency? Or all of the above?

13. When buying wax should I ask about the number of purges it underwent? Should I buy a pricey wax just because a budtender tells me its good or should I ask if they had it tested and how it was made? Local or imported?

14. When buying hash oil, should I ask about how it was made and from what? For example, what parts of the plant were used? The fan leaf trim and stems? The popcorn sized buds? The premium or choice buds from the plant? Or the shake from stored pounds of old harvest?

15. Should I have a maximum amount I'm willing to spend on hash oil or should I spend what it costs to stay medicated?

16. Should I relocate to a state with tolerance if my needs can't be met safely in my state? Is it worth going to prison for medicating for my condition or should I move?

17. Is my condition treatable with medical marijuana? If so, should I try

other medicines first or consult my tolerant physician about using medical marijuana?

18. Am I ashamed of having to rely on medical marijuana due to my political beliefs or job title? If so, how does my right to privacy impact my choices about which clubs can address my needs around protecting my use of medical marijuana? Should I opt for delivery based clubs or do I need community support?

19. Does my job drug test? How do I navigate around my need for medical marijuana versus my employer's right to fire me for failing a urinalysis? How do I inform an employer about my being a compliant medical marijuana patient? What do I do if they fire me for failing a urinalysis after producing a Doctor's note?

20. How do I handle running into people from my private, work, or social circle when medicated?

21. If I am not into crafting concentrates, buying an Omicron, or haggling with clubs but want to try vaporizing instead of combustion, which device sounds right for me? Should I opt for

an Arizer with a glass stem? Should I
go for a plastic, tough NO2 by Vapir
that can be used on the charger or
has a battery for short excursions?
Should I look into the Magic Flight
Launch Box for durability and
portability? Should I consider a
butane powered vape like the Iolite?
Should I consider an Essential Vape
for concentrates and flowers?

22. Should I ask clubs about where they
get their medicine? Is the club a free
for all that buys anything that walks
in the door? Do they test their buds?
Do they test their concentrates? Do
they grow the medicine on site or in
the community or is it brought in from
anywhere? If so, is the method used
to bring it to me legal or am I at risk
for possessing it, even with a note
from my Doctor?

23. Did my purchase help support a club
with sound environmental and ethical
practices? Did my purchase help
finance a shaky, shady club with
loose rules and medicine from
vendors who are involved in hard
drug sales and/or abuse?

24. If I stop coming to a club can I
request that my personal information

be destroyed or expunged from their data storage? How long do clubs hang on to my personal information if I only go once or relocate?

25. When traveling to other states or countries with no tolerance for medical marijuana, how will I meet my needs? Will I call ahead to the airport? Will I produce my paperwork and medical marijuana upon arriving at the airport? Can I be arrested or detained at my local airport for possessing medical marijuana even if I have my paperwork?

Choosing your medication based on your symptom(s):

When choosing strains, it is important to select one that best meets your needs. Indicas tend to be more powerful than Sativas. Sativas have less chlorophyll, higher THC content to CBD ratios, and offer a vibrant buzz with less sedation. Sativas are thought to function as an antidepressant for some patients and as creative fuel for others. Sativas are thought to tackle mild headaches and migraines. They are also believed to reduce awareness of intensity of pain for chronic pain patients. Sativas may reduce nausea and stimulate the appetite. Indicas have a higher CBD to THC ratio when compared to Sativas. Indicas are believed to possess anxiolytic properties. CBD has been used as an anticonvulsant and to reduce edema. Some patients find relief from pain, spasms, tremor, bradykinesia, tardive dyskinesia, and bruxism. Some patients report relief from insomnia, pressure inside the eye, and nausea/appetite disturbance. Some patients report a reduction in seizure frequency which results in an overall increase in seizure threshold from use of high CBD strains.

A statement about the need for solid, empirical evidence for using medical marijuana:

Marijuana has been here and been used by man since antiquity. This does not mean we know everything about it. The truth and platform used by antimarijuana forces is that we simply do not know enough about marijuana to say if it is useful or applicable to the diseases and conditions it is meant to treat. We lack a solid body of replicable research with adequate sample sizes and airtight research designed to isolate the variables we believe marijuana impacts with use. We know next to nothing about proper dose interval and opt to medicate at will. The average medicating consumer applies their medical marijuana whenever they feel symptoms returning which can be a slippery slope when considering iatrogenically induced addiction/addictive behaviors. Patients left to medicate at will gives the medical marijuana movement less credibility. It is vital for us to provide replicable data from long term, well funded studies meant to isolate and regulate the smallest, most effective dose that does the least amount of harm to the patient and isolates their symptom constellation. If we continue to push to allow patients to medicate at will by simply providing them with semi-legal access to medical marijuana and doctors who will sign them off for a fee, we will fail at displaying the true potential and power of this life giving plant. Help find and finance research for real applications of medical marijuana.

The Omicron and Pure Gold hash oil were chosen as the best working examples of a viable anticarcinogenic means to an end. The Omicron provides a safer vehicle to medicating than combustion powered devices and features reloadable cartridges. The Omicron meters doses of whatever concentrate the patient has loaded. The metered vape hits last as long as six seconds. The Pure Gold hash oil has been crafted using isomesmerization, is tested for purity and potency, and is mass produced to meet the needs of a demanding, growing medicating consumer population. Together, the Omicron loaded with Pure Gold represents the future of vaporizing with medical marijuana. Now, the task is to study, create or refine strains for specific diagnoses, and design concentrates to address specific symptoms. Patients of the future will be able to select strains, a dosing regiment, and device for vaporizing based on empirically validated, replicable findings from well funded research. Until then, enjoy vaporizing with medical marijuana! And, please do what ever you can to help finance or support research efforts.

Thanks to the Purple Elephant Co-op for having the best deal on the Pure Gold used to research this book. Visit them online at: purpleelephantcoop.com If you are in San Francisco, try this delivery service's hash oil: thegreencross.org

Vaporizing Medical Marijuana II: The Omicron & Arizer Solo Portable Boogaloo!

Vaping is like getting into a boogaloo or groovy dance. Once you pop, you can't stop. Omicron vaporizers have revolutionized vaping as we know it. This follow up to my Bestselling ebook "Vaporizing Medical Marijuana" (included) was a necessity as soon as I discovered the Omicron online. I knew my ebook that was released in October of this year, 2011, was made virtually obsolete by the emergence of this technology. After careful research and consideration, I selected the Omicron pen sized vaporizer due to its portability and refillable cartridge. There are many other fine pen vapes on the market. If you are in an area where refill medicine is in constant supply, try one. The Omicron offers vaping of oils to people world wide. I'm going to tell you how to make your own concentrates to load into your cartridges. But, I must first define and outline some key concepts and priniciples to using the Omicron and Arizer Solo in conjunction. There are those of us who just can't or won't say goodbye to our love of flowers. The Arizer Solo is the best way to taste them. But, did you know your Arizer works in perfect harmony with your Omicron? That's right. I made a discovery worth writing an entire book about. The Arizer heats anything. Therefore, it can be used to get your semi-solid concentrates into liquid form for refilling your Omicron cartridge! I'm going to teach you how. If you are sampling this ebook for free, please consider purchasing before reading on. It costs less than a buck. If you are borrowing this on Prime, thank you. Now, let's cut right to the chase: what is the goal of medicating?

The Goal of medicating with Marijuana is to acheive the best, longest lasting effect with the least amount of harm to our bodies.

Therefore, if we select the purest, strongest form of THC and consolidate the method of administration to minimize physical harm, we have won. We have the future in our hands. I'm going to illustrate how using the Arizer and

Omicron can reshape your view on medicating. Some of the traditional methods are going to be discussed. We embrace all medicators and beliefs but let's face facts together: old methods are carcinogenic. I have proof. Look at your old glass bong. Chances are the residue coated densely around and inside it and the components is difficult to remove. Imagine the inside of your body next time you gawk at that dirty bong or glass piece. What makes you think there isn't a similar but impossible to clean build up inside of you? Tetrahydrocannabinol delta 9 is water soluble. Some argue that the lungs cleanse the build up by breaking it down. I cannot confirm this but more importantly they have left out a critical factor: tar. Tar comes from the burning of leafy matter. There is no escaping it. If you use combustion to smoke or accidentally combust medicine by vaping at too high of a temperature, you are getting tar. I don't need a panel of scientists to warn me that tar causes cancer. It is already printed on every pack of cigarettes in the world. How different could burning a dry, leafy product be? I don't care to find out. If you wish to stick with combustion be my guest but this ebook won't advocate potentially carcinogenic methods of medicating. Do I medicate with a joint once in a while? Sure! But, the taste of vaping has ruined even the top shelf flowers. So, be forewarned. If you switch to the Arizer and Omicron method, you won't like combusting like you used to. Using the Arizer to vape flowers is sufficient to last a lifetime with the utmost preservation of flavor profiles in most hits. But, the Omicron takes vaping to the highest level imaginable. Medicators can now vape extremely potent concentrates. The Arizer and all methods before it are obsolete. Dabbers will be upset at my revelation but my question to any dabber is how do you know you are getting vapes when your temperature varies so greatly? Please feel free to educate me and I love you, brothers and sisters who dab, but are you concerned about heat regulation or consistency? Is that dab not smoking or is that vape? And, how do you accout for portability? Dabbing requires components that seem less portable. If I am wrong or have stepped on any toes, I apologize. But, I will state that I have never dabbed before so I cannot speak from experience. Maybe I will come to Colorado and write a third book on alternate methods of medicating with concentrates? For now, suffice it to say that in my estimation the Omicron wears the crown.

Let's find out how:

1. Potency- Concentrates can be used. Therefore, any flower that tests lower than any concentrate in THC can't compare. The medicine used is more potent than any used in any flower vaporizer or hash pipe on the market. Hash pipes use combustion. Hash is wasted during combustion. Vaping oil or other semi-solids assures full use of medicine bought. Potency cannot be discussed without discussing the cost effective ways used to medicate. A vape that stretches a gram of hash oil out for hundreds of hits cannot be compared with any other method for that reason alone. Think about it: You spend tons of money on flowers to stay medicated but the potency is lacking, in comparison to medicating with concentrates. Therefore, would

it not make more sense to buy a liquid or semi-solid form of medical marijuana that can be vaped longer and is exponentially stronger? Why not purchase the Trippy stick or any glycerine bound concentrate cartridge vaporizer? The Omicron does not require a third party. You can bypass the club. Clubs are going to make money off of you by forcing you to buy a new prefilled cartridge each time you run out. With the Omicron, buy or make your own oil or semi-solid. If your club closes or you move, you won't be stuck with a vape you can't use. Therefore, potency and cost effectiveness of the Omicron outshines all other pipes, vaporizers, and methods for medicating, except (possibly) consumption.

2.   No need for combustion powered heating device- Some vapes on the market use a regular lighter to heat a concentrate. Some use a small or large torch to heat for medicating with concentrates. Some vapes run off of reloadable tanks of combustible gases. This third industry benefits. The Omicron has

made all of them obsolete due to the implementation of the rechargeable battery. The only vape that might remain valid is the Essential Vape. Why? Because it allows the medicator to vape hash in a glass vial. But, the potency may not reach that of a semi-solid, liquid, butane honey oil, CO_2 extract, taffy, or wax. So, medicators must revisit the "Potency" argument to decide if the Essential Vape is worthy of your quiver. I have not tried one yet and it sounds like book three has another potential chapter. So, forget about any other vape that needs heat. The only heat source you need is to reload cartridges. You aren't inhaling it. Its just liquifying concentrate into the cartridge.

3.   Size- The Omicron's size, power, potency, portability, cost effectiveness, and refillable cartridge make it a stand alone vape. This Sharpee-sized pen vape Is ultra-discrete. The size is right for the discrete medicator on the go or the traveler. If you think the Omicron's size means it can only be used as directed I have great news for you. It

has a Bubbler attachment in development. And, like the Arizer with an O-ring on it, the Omicron can be used on your bong. Don't go direct. Tube it. Why? Putting a tube from the Omicron directly into the bong allows you to use the Omicron as a carb. I attempted to go mouthpiece to female stem with ice water in my sparkling clean bong with success. I recommend thick oil in your cartridge or semi-solids when tilting to take hits. Viscosity factors in to clogging. I find that "upright is alright." Why? Because keeping your Omicron upright at all times but especially when hitting is key to keeping airflow maximized. Think: you are dealing with a liquid. Observe that vial of hash oil you got. Notice how it collects on the bottom. Our old friend gravity keeps the sludged goodness hugging the bottom. That is its natural state. Cartridges left on their sides lend themselves to clogging as gravity will move the liquid inside lengthwise. You can do anything with the battery piece. But by all means keep your carts upright to allow gravity to be your ally not your enemy! Size and future attachments and the use of a tube to attach to your bong adds the Omicron another jewel to its Corona of features. Small but vapable through water. And, its more potent. Size also ties into durability. The small stainless steel Omicron won't shatter. Flavor is not compromised just as gas isn't wasted in your engine. You want efficiency and durability plus small size. This is the Omicron's secret weapon. It has all three.

4. Most cost effective versus all other methods- Vaping hash oil or other semi-solids seems expensive. In researching the investment, I concluded that my love of vaping flowers was worth retaining and then I discovered the Arizer works with the Omicron. I now think every medicator who loves flowers but who needs cost effective medicating should invest in an Arizer and an Omicron. Why? The Arizer can be used to get concentrate heated for placement into the Omicron cartridge via a glass dropper. Therefore, you have a way to enjoy flowers and

prep oils for loading into Omicron cartridges. The one-two punch combo is sure to win over the biggest skeptics and traditional combustion medicators. Flowers used in the Arizer can be retained and made into butter (recipe included below). Or, you can use your Arizer to liquify concentrates. I prefer both. The cost of a cartridge which yields hundreds of hits versus daily over combustion using traditional methods is tiny. If you still enjoy vaping flowers, you can retain them after vaping for cooking when using the Arizer. Medicators who combine the Arizer and Omicron never waste medicine or money. The Arizer offers a way to reload on the go also by liquifying concentrates with ease.

5. Portability & durability- The Omicron and Arizer could fit in one pocket, without cases. The Omicron is stainless steel and is impervious to most damage, except water. The Omicron lasts as long as the battery life and medicator allow. The Arizer comes with a glass tube or diffuser. The glass is thick but not

shatterproof. The Omicron offers another layer to portability by allowing medicators to charge it via USB from their USB port on any device. There is also a car charger adapter.

6.   Accessories- The Omicron firmly grasps the medicating consumer by the lapels by offering a vast array of accessories. Some are in development, like the Bubbler attachment. Others are available now, like the Adapters that allow medicators to vape any atomizer or cartridge. The Adapter set has 510, 808, and 901 sized adapters for all other carts. Now, you can enjoy any size or try any preloaded cart from any club. The inventor of the Omicron warns users that carts bound with glycerine are limited in potency. He also advises users to consider vaping with pure concentrate to get the strongest effect. Carts that use cotton and glycerine or any combination of binding chemicals to produce vapor fall far short of the mark and cannot be compared to loading pure concentrate. Most of the vapor

produced appears to be loaded with THC and tastes great, some are even flavored, but the truth is medicators are limiting themselves due to the chemical reality that diluted or bound THC cannot be compared to vaping pure concentrate with no additives. Other accessories include: an adapter for charging in the car, a filling tool that covers the airtube for ease of loading, back up chargers, a master case of carts, and a warranty on the battery that lasts one year from receipt date. Other vapes do not offer warranties and if a consumer gets a faulty one, they are stuck with it. Why? Because you can't ship it if it has had any contact with your medical marijuana. You risk committing a felony by mailing it back to the manufacturer. The Omicron stands behind their product by offering an iron clad warranty on the battery.

7. Discretion and ease of use- Not all medicators can vape as freely as they choose. Some must remain hidden. The Omicron has answered countless prayers from the discrete

medicator. Not only does it come to life and produce rich potent vapor in seconds, it fits neatly in one's pocket right after vaping. Ducking and dodging to avoid the Law or nosey family used to mean stealth missions to the nether regions of the yard or garage. Not anymore. The Omicron gives the discrete medicator free reign over when and where they medicate. Ease of use means no waiting to vape. Even the mighty Arizer takes minutes to heat flowers and after each vape must go through a refractory heating period. The Omicron offers back to back hits until either the battery dies or the cart dies, whichever comes first. Ease of use means no prep time either. For all other vapes, medicators must prep, which takes time. With the Arizer, medicators must take time to grind flower, wait for device to heat, load glass piece, and wait again for flowers to heat up before vaping. The Omicron needs seconds. All other vapes need minutes or trap you with non-refillable carts. Having a refillable cart with adapters to vape any cart or atomizer, sets the

Omicron so far apart from competitors it renders them obsolete.

8. Technology and practical design plus refillable carts with rechargeable battery- The Omicron brings technology right to your fingertips with the push of a button. Medicators who are married to the past and use combustion will attempt to find fault with the Omicron and will fall short. There is no comparison when considering the overall practicality, potency, portability, anticarcinogenic, and efficiency factors. By offering medicators a new way to relieve symptoms in seconds using the purest, most potent medicine in liquid or semi-solid state from a dose regulating device that offers refillable cartridges and a rechargeable battery, the Omicron leaves everybody else in the dust. If you think that's impossible, I have more news to disrupt your paradigm. The Inventor of the Omicron is releasing several new Vaporizers that hold multiple carts, use different battery configurations, and boast carts with upwards of nine-hundred hits. The only person to make the Omicron

seem outdated or too small is the Inventor! He is beating his competitors to the punch by creating more Vaporizers that put him on his own tier. Think of how many people around the world suffering from symptoms that can be relieved with medical marijuana are going to benefit from this one man's invention. I think he should be given huge, global praise and recognition for developing a device potentially as useful as a shot for patients with Wasting syndrome, Cancer, AIDS, spasticity, cerebral palsy, appetite disturbance, PTSD, nausea, depression, anxiety, and countless other bodily or spiritual woes that can turn fatal. The Omicron and its Inventor are saviors, from a medical perspective. I look forward to seeing how much these vaporizers will reshape the medical marijuana industry as we know it. Did I mention I think THC Scientific should be nominated for best invention for treating with medical marijuana? Okay. I've voiced my opinion. Now, its your turn to test it out.

Finding and buying your Omicron and accessories plus tips:

You can find an Omicron in seconds by searching online. Shop around for best shipping prices. The Omicron now comes in three different finishes. The newest Vaporizer by the same Inventor of the Omicron is called the Persei. I look forward to including details about it in book three. I would imagine the Persei to be the best vaporizer on the market now, including the Omicron. Why? Because the Persei offers the same benefits times two and various battery configurations for more control of your doses. Other vaporizers in development from the Omicron family include: the Eight, the Alpha, and the Centauri. For now, I am going to focus on the Omicron as the Persei is not sitting right in front of me..yet. I paid less than one-hundred and fifty for my two Omicrons with one cart. The kit came with a sturdy case inscribed with the Omicron name. Each battery says "Omicron" on it. The cartridge comes with a rubber mouthpiece and cap. There is also a sleeve to protect fingers from hot battery or cart. The sleeve slides on and screws into place. The charger is versatile in that it can be plugged into any USB port or plug. The filling tool is sometimes included for free on the company website for THC Scientific. They are currently available on delta9vapes dot com. The filling tool is designed to cover the air tube hole to allow medicine to fill carts with ease and no mess. If you want to be able to vape any cart or atomizer, buy the adapter set. I also suggest buying a five pack of empty carts. Why? Because you may want to have a few different carts around for variety. Vaping the same oil or semi-solid everyday creates a tolerance, much like one develops when vaping the same flowers day in, day out. Keeping a variety of carts with different medicines allows medicators constant relief and a varied experience instead of a uniform one dictated and limited by tolerance. The other downside to developing a tolerance to stronger and stronger concentrates is it takes more and more to get relief from symptoms. I encourage heavy medicators to revisit how they can acheive daily relief by adding variety to their carts instead of filling all of them with the same concentrate. Buy extra carts and if you are in the car enough, buy the car adapter. Please don't drive while medicating or medicated. You just get in the way. And, in California, you can be issued a DUI, even if you have your medical marijuana paperwork and state card. Don't medicate while driving or medicate then drive. The car charger is for responsible use only. Don't give medicating or medicators a bad reputation by getting arrested for medicating while driving or in your car. Some medicators may want to buy an extra charger to have on hand. Others may wish to check back online for new releases in accessories, like the Bubbler. You will also need to buy a regular lighter or small torch lighter for use in refilling your carts. You will also need to buy a glass eye-dropper, if you are going to use hash oil and my Arizer method to reload your carts. Do not buy or use plastic droppers. Why? Plastic may leech into heated concentrate or the plastic tube may react by melting or changing shape under heat. The outcome could be squirting expensive hash oil all over the place or melting the tip of the dropper by trying to draw heated concentrates in or push them out. All unwanted outcomes can be avoided by avoiding plastics. Always use glass. You might want to purchase vice grips or a C-clamp to hold carts upright for refilling. Don't grip the cart bottom too tight. Use just enough pressure to hold it steady while refilling. If you are purchasing hash oil from a club, keep the vials if they are glass. That way, if your club closes or you move or have to make your own concentrates, you have glass to keep it in. Never depend solely on clubs or dispensaries if your condition requires daily medicating. I advise you to learn how to grow your own medicine using my method (included below) and make your own concentrates. Medicators who depend on clubs are at a disadvantage when compared with self-sustaining medicators who can produce their own medicine and craft their own concentrates. The only other piece of equipment I recommend is a clicker to count hits. You should keep track of exactly how many doses or hits you are getting from whatever type of concentrate you load. Over time, you will discover lower viscosity concentrates or semi-solids (earwax, taffy, CO_2 extract, butane honey oil, pure gold) provide the most relief per cartridge. Careful medicators can select just the right consistency and quality for their needs per cartridge per day. You can reclaim control over dosing, unlike wasteful over combustion of flowers or hash or kief which leads to mixed day-to-day results and overspending/overconsumption to stave off symptoms. Regulate dosing with the Omicron or overspend on medicating.

Finding and buying the Arizer Solo and using it with the Omicron plus tips:

The Arizer Solo can also be found online for half price in seconds. I wouldn't pay more than one-hundred and fifty dollars for it. Shop around to see who has the best bundle deals or shipping prices but don't pay full retail, unless you want to spend three-hundred bucks on something you can get for half price. The Arizer comes with two glass mouthpieces for vaping and a critical third piece for my method: a glass bowl piece for heating oils. This critical third piece of glass is thrown in with the

Arizer to market it for aromatherapy. We all know the truth is they had to mask its real purpose, medicating with marijuana. So, now that I have outted them, let's go over how to use the Arizer to liquify oils to use in your Omicron cartridges. If you want to use the Arizer to vape flowers, please read on. The instructions are in book one, included with this ebook.

<u>How to use the Arizer Solo to liquify Hash oil to load an Omicron cartridge:</u>

You will need the following items to load using this method:

1.   The Omicron pen vape and all included components.
2.   The Arizer Solo portable and the glass bowl piece included with it.
3.   A lighter or torch lighter. Do not overheat any components during this process.
4.   Glass eye-dropper with small opening. Wide droppers are messy.
5. A vial of one gram of hash oil. Do not load more than a gram.
6.   A toothpick to lightly place in the air hole tube in the Omicron cartridge.

7.   Vice grips or a C-clamp to hold
cartridge firmly in place while
loading.

Step-by-step guide to filling the Omicron
using the Arizer as a heating element:

1.   Select a large, adequate surface
area to load cartridges. Keep all
drinks and any other items that are
not needed out of the way. Do not
clutter loading area.
2.   Start by securing the bottom of the
cartridge with the vice grips or
clamp. Be careful not to grip too
tight. Make sure cartridge is clear by
inspecting it before clamping. This is
done by screwing the empty
cartridge onto the battery and
pressing the button. If cartridge is
good, you will see an orange glow
when viewing from the top through
the air tube hole. If you do not see
an orange light, cartridge may be
compromised or unusable. Do not
attempt to load cartridges that fail the
glow test.
3.   If your cart passes the glow test,
secure it at the base and observe the
state your hash oil is in. Is your hash

oil in a glass vial? If yes, test the vial to see if it will fit snugly in the chamber of the Arizer. If so, turn the Arizer on. Turn the heat up to "1" on the temperature dial. Allow the Arizer to heat up all the way before inspecting oil. If the hash oil is still solid, turn the temperature up on the Arizer to "2" and observe oil as it is heating up. Do not overheat hash oil. It will vaporize the THC inside. Do not turn heat up past "2" in haste to liquify the hash oil. You will end up vaping it. Watch the vial by pulling it out every few seconds to see when it has liquified completely. Vial will get hot but not too hot to handle, if so temp down.

4. Heat the top 1/4 of the cartridge before attempting to load it. Why? Heat must be present for the liquid to slide down and into the cartridge. You heat by passing the torch or lighter by the cartridge's top 1/4 portion for no more than two seconds at a time per side. Do not overheat top in haste. There are delicate seals inside the cartridge. You risk compromising them by overheating. Use the toothpick to

plug the air tube hole lightly while loading. You may place it now. Grab your glass eye-dropper also. You are ready to load.

5.   Allow the Arizer enough time to heat up and liquify your hash oil before using the glass eye-dropper to pull it out and load into the slits on the side of the Omicron cartridge. Work fast and stop to heat up top 1/4 of cartridge after every squirt. Load the entire gram. Do not try to load more than one gram. Simply fill another cartridge.

6.   Once you have filled the cartridge, switch off the Arizer. Allow it and the cartridge a few minutes to cool off. Be sure to place the plastic storage cap (included) snugly onto the cartridge if you are storing. Leave it off for immediate use. Do not bypass the cooling off period. It is vital to cartridge longevity and efficiency.

7.   If your hash oil vial does not fit the Arizer chamber itself simply use the included glass bowl piece. Vials or the concentrate itself can be placed in the glass bowl piece. The temperature will be increased to make up for the distance from the

heat source and this means you must underline observe carefully and test temperature to make sure it doesn't get too hot. Use your fingertips to gauge heat. Watch for changes in the concentrate's consistency and viscosity. Lean over the heating concentrate and smell it. It should smell like marijuana not burnt popcorn. If it smells like its cooking, it is. Do not overheat concentrates, you will vaporize the THC. Once it has liquified, pull it into the dropper and load cartridge using the same method described above. If you are having difficulty getting all of the concentrate out of the dropper, simply heat it well above where the concentrate is positioned. The heat will cause it to liquify and drip out the tip. Do not overheat to attempt to get every molecule of it. It is impossible. I have burned fingertips to prove it. Heat is only used sparingly in every facet of this process. Overheating will cause more problems than you can imagine and waste expensive concentrate. Do not overheat the cartridge or any portion below the top 1/4 of it. The instructions for refilling overemphasize not overheating. I am doing my best to warn you and avoid bad reviews from those who rushed the process. Do not overheat items used in refilling. The filling tool is no exception. To use it, you place it over the cartridge, load your concentrate or vial upside down, and heat it into the cartridge. Again, use heat sparingly and only hold heat source close to cartridge or filling tool for a maximum of two seconds. Any more than that and you risk overheating and zapping all the THC. Don't let your stoke to medicate make you overheat or speed up the process to start vaping before cart cools off completely. You read it here and you will see it in the user's guide, <u>do</u> <u>not</u> overheat.

<u>Vaping with the Omicron:</u>

Once your cartridge has had time to cool off, it is time to test it out. Start by making sure your Omicron is fully charged. Carefully remove the plastic cap from the cartridge and screw it onto the battery. Keep the Omicron vertical for best hits. Remember: you are vaping liquid from a small cylinder through an air hole tube. Tilting the Omicron horizontally will also tilt the liquid inside once its heated. This may or may not effect hit quality. However, I find the Omicron to hit best vertically. Screw the sleeve on then the rubber mouthpiece. It is time to take your first pull. Press and hold the button for exactly six seconds while slowly sipping vapor into your mouth, not your lungs. After drawing for six seconds, release the button but continue to draw. Why? Because you are keeping the air hole tube clear by continuing to draw after your hit. Once vapor has entered the oral cavity, draw it deep into the lungs using your breath, after removing the Omicron from your lips. Do not "power hit" the Omicron in an effort to draw vapor deep into the lungs. You risk clogging it. Think of the cylinder as having a little bong stem inside. What happens when you pull too hard on a bong? You get a big mouth full of bong water as punishment. Your Omicron works the same way. The air hole tube is like a straw sticking in a pool of hash oil. If you hit it just right, you get vapors. Too much and you force liquid up the tube that will lead to clogging. If your cartridge clogs, refer to the included guide to unclogging that came with the kit. I have not had any clogging issues perhaps due to proper loading of the cartridge, not overheating, not pulling too hard, and using well made concentrate. I have experienced the "pop" reported by many users. The "pop" is when hitting the cartridge for the first time at room temperature. Sometimes, the cartridge needs just enough heat to free up the semi-solid to be vaped. When holding down the button for six seconds, it is not uncommon to feel the pop then experience a robust vapor. There are specific instructions on how to prime cartridges that are not drawing. I will refer you to those for troubleshooting type questions. The Omicron cartridge and the various concentrates used present a challenge to medicators to find which ones work best and provide the most relief. I encourage readers to search forums online for tips and advice. If your unable to use your Omicron, contact the manufacturer. I am not liable for any damage to or loss of product for imparting these suggestions. This is merely my own opinion of what I found works best when pairing the Arizer with the Omicron. My suggestions and experience with both the Arizer and Omicron are independent of the manufacturer or any other group, club, or user.

Making your own concentrates:

Butane Honey Oil (BHO)

1. Search online for an extractor tube for making BHO. You can also craft them out of various materials. Search videos online for how to make your own if you do not wish to buy one. Most videos use a piece of PVC pipe with capped ends. People drill five holes in one cap and one hole in the other.
2. Load the extractor tube with the highest quality shake you can find or afford. Most extractor tubes hold at least an ounce. Once tube is loaded, insert the thrice refined butane into the end and depress. Be sure to buy the most refined butane you can find, make sure it has been refined at

least three times. It will say it on the bottle.

3.   You will be spraying the butane through the extractor tube and into a large rectangular Pyrex dish. As the butane makes its way down the extractor tube, it will get cold. Be sure to have a towel over it or risk burning your fingers. Allow all of the butane to drain through the extractor tube and into the Pyrex dish. This process must be done outdoors far away from anything flammable. Once the butane has emptied, the liquid in the Pyrex will bubble. Allow bubbles to form but be sure to pop them with a razor if they dry. There is flammable gas inside each unpopped bubble. Pop them all. Once byproduct has dried, scrape it with a razor and smear onto parchment. Allow product to sit at least twenty-four hours before using.

4.   Most medicators will want to refine their BHO by vacuum purging it. Vacuum purging removes flammables by placing the BHO in a vacuum that removes oxygen. There are plenty of videos online on how to purge. I recommend viewing all of

them and deciding on which method fits your budget. Purging is highly recommended. I would not consume any Butane-based cannabis product that hadn't been purged several times, just to be safe. Using expensive, refined butane won't guarantee impurities are all gone. Vacuum purging zaps them for sure. Repeated purging just makes BHO better. Cruise youtube, you'll see.

CO2 Extract:

1.	You will need a 22-micron hash making bag, at least an ounce of shake, and two blocks of dry ice. Begin by crushing the dry ice with a mallet into chunks. Dry ice is cold enough to burn flesh. Be mindful of that when working with it. Never touch it. Always place a barrier between your skin and dry ice. Once you have smashed it down, add it to the 22-micron bag. Add all the shake to the bag and mix with dry ice. Place a pyrex dish underneath the mesh portion of the hash making bag with the dry ice and shake inside.

2. Vigorously shake the bag with the mesh portion remaining over the dish. Continue to shake as hard as you can until nothing comes out and into the dish. This may take several minutes. Once the byproduct hits the dish, the atmospheric pressure acts to purge it of impurities. Once it has stopped "smoking" the CO_2 extract can be refined further. For more on how to refine CO_2 extract, search videos online. You will need to select the method that best suits your budget and expertise.

Note: for both of the above stated methods, I am in no way liable or responsible for any unwanted outcomes or wasted medicine from using these methods. Readers are being advised right here, right now, that using Butane or Dry Ice could be hazardous to their health. Never use Butane or make BHO indoors. That is just stupid. Watch out for smokers if you are outdoors. One spark and you could do like Cheech and Chong and go up in smoke yourself. Butane and dry ice are dangerous. Use caution and research both thoroughly before attempting these techniques.

These suggestions were only put in place for readers who cannot acquire concentrates and must make their own.

Have fun, be sure to purge and refine. But, most of all stay safe.

This concludes book two. Below is book one which includes instructions on using the Arizer to vape flowers. It also includes instructions on how to grow your own and a butter recipe for post-vaporized flower. I hope you've enjoyed reading and learning about vaporizing medical marijuana! Stay tuned for book three, coming soon!

Dedicated to: The Green Cross for always being there and taking care of me during my illness. Thanks a million! I would also like to thank THC Scientific, Inc. for developing such a revolutionary vaporizer. Enjoy vaporizing and reducing cancer!

Vaporizing Medical Marijuana #1
Bestseller (Book One)

Medical Marijuana versus Acquired Marijuana

This comparative analysis is intended for patients who are prescribed Medical Marijuana. The vaporizers selected bypass combustion by heating the crumbled marijuana flowers thereby making them anticarcinogenic. Vapor is hot and may cause respiratory irritation. Patients may cough or experience lung or throat irritation. Vapor is from convection. Combustion produces a tar which is believed to be carcinogenic. The truth is science has not researched medical applications of marijuana to the extent they would other more toxic treatments. Most of us accept that marijuana causes hunger. Being hungry leads to eating. Eating leads to weight gain for patients suffering from wasting syndrome. Therefore, one clear example of a life saving application of medical marijuana warrants this book. Vaporizers offer a safer alternative for patients who cannot ingest marijuana without adverse or unwanted outcomes. Some patients have no choice but to inhale to get medicated. Vaporizers use convection to eliminate the tars. There is no wasted medicine. The medical marijuana from the vaporizer can be retained and used to make edibles. Heat from convection is believed to zap most cannabinoids. Some cannabinoids remain and with several ounces of quantity, they can be cooked into butter and any other variation of edible. Unlike combustion, convection simply browns the crumbled marijuana flowers. For all vaporizers compared, I invite patients to see them as ovens. The temperatures are similar to your oven at home. For example, if you want toast to be light brown, you don't broil it. On all vaporizers compared, the lowest effective convection temperature is preferred. With the Magic Flight Launch Box, the patient must control the temperature by applying pressure to the removable, rechargable battery. On the Arizer Solo, the temperature is toggled up and down from one to seven. On the two Vapir models, the temperature is displayed digitally. Both Vapir models feature toggling buttons, up and down.

Heating your medicine is a fine art. Achieving full extraction is the goal. Taste, effect, and other variables will be considered. Medicating is nothing to be ashamed of for law abiding patients in tolerant states or countries. If you are medicating, lift yourself up above any shame. Let medical marijuana heal you. It will. This guide is not for users who acquired marijuana without a prescription. Patients should address questions about the products discussed to their respective manufacturers and their prescribing physician. The idea behind this analysis is to teach by comparison how basic types of vaporizers can be used by patients. Three of the vaporizers offer portability for the patient on the go. The Vapir bag inflatable plugs in. All of the vaporizers discussed will be presented in terms of their strengths. All four are great for medicating patients. There are hundreds of vaporizers available online and in retail. I selected these four vaporizers based on there construction, quality, and vapor volume. Purchase any or all of them if your are medicating. You can't go wrong.

Your Guide

John Mayer announced to the media his cancellation of the remainder of his tour dates due to a granuloma on his vocal cord. I have the same thing. I am also a writer. I have tons of fiction and nonfiction. If you like this book, try some of my other stuff. I wrote a lot while I was on vocal rest. For those of you who may not know, vocal rest means no talking. I literally was not allowed to speak for three months. My granuloma shrunk over time. I used prescribed medical marijuana to treat my benign tumor. I cannot attribute the reduction in size entirely to vaporizing as vocal rest is probably more responsible. I smoked medical marijuana at first before opting to vaporize to reduce carcinogens, preserve medicine, and improve flavor profiles. On my journey, I invested over five hundred dollars in these four devices based on the reviews and videos I watched. I wanted to take a break from fiction writing and share this important information with other patients. Having a condition amenable to medical marijuana isn't always good news. My condition is treatable with lasic surgery if vocal rest fails. Other patients have dismal diagnoses. I want to send a special message of hope and love to you. If you are battling a difficult or life threatening illness or condition, I wish you all the best. I worked in hospice for years. I am a Neuropsychologist. I wrote this for you and others who may benefit from vaporizing medical marijuana when it cannot be ingested.

Vaporizers compared:

1. The Vapir Digital Air bag inflatable with optional whip and mouthpiece-

This vaporizer retails for around $120.00. The box includes bags, the whip, screens, cleaning brush, extra tubing, and the Digital Air device itself. Paitents need to know they must purchase the stand if they do not wish to hold the device upright while medicating. It includes a wrist strap.

2. The Magic Flight Launch Box-

This is the most compact vaporizer. It retails for around $100.00. The box includes a storage tin with logo, a brush, two rechargable AA batteries and charger, two mouthpieces, two rubberbands to secure the sliding lid while transporting, and a black velvet drawstring bag. An adapter is available for patients who prefer to plug in when near an electrical outlet.

3. The Vapir NO2 Portable Lithium-Ion battery powered Vaporizer-

This vaporizer offers patients the ability to plug in or travel. The NO2 retails for around $180.00. The box includes the device, two bamboo stirring tools, a cleaning brush, screens, mouthpieces, extra tubing, and charger. Extra batteries are available and swap out from the bottom.

4. The Arizer Solo Portable Vaporizer-

The Arizer brings glass on ceramic to the Patient. For maximum flavor extraction, glass on glass wears the crown in the taste kingdom. The Arizer is the flavor king of the bunch. The battery life outlasts all current comparable models. It cannot be used while plugged in but an adapter is available for Patients who want to medicate in the car or from an electrical outlet. The Arizer retails from $150.00 to $300.00. Patients are encouraged to search online or in retail for fair prices on the Arizer.

Selecting Medical Marijuana

Before I discuss the vaporizers, I felt it was prudent to discuss medication. Let's keep it simple and stick with the two major types: Indicas and Sativas. I recommend strong Indicas. I find Indicas to be far more therapeutic in there range of effects. In Northern California, Purple strains are popular due to there fruity flavor profiles and purple flowers. Patients find them to be sedating. Most patients report a marked increase in their appetites. Strain varietals are vast and beyond the scope of this book. I would make the following suggestions when selecting medication:

1. Get medical marijuana that comes from a legal club that tests their strains. Most quality cannabis clubs test their strains for pesticides, molds, bugs, and pass the medicine under an ultraviolet light to kill any remaining mold and bugs. Don't bother with clubs who don't test their medicine. Medicine should be thoroughly examined before being given to patients. Remember: you can eat the browned flowers left from

vaporizing. If you plan on eating or vaporizing a strain, make sure you know it is clean.

2. Find a club that tests the THC content. The perk to testing strains for pesticides, molds, and bugs is most clubs get THC content profiles. Indicas with higher than 17% are effective and usually more flavorful. Sativas and hybrids are great for patients who need less sedating effects but most patients find the sedative effects function as an anxiolytic. If you are sensitive to medicating, look for Indica strains that offer flavor with modest 12-16% THC content.

3. Invest in a quality metal grinder. Plastic and wood grinders invariably sheer off in tiny pieces into your medicine during grinding. Quality metal grinders do not sheer. When grinding medical marijuana flowers for using any of these four vaporizers, do not overgrind. That is, grinding into a coarse powder is preferable to a fine powder. Fine powder ground medical marijuana flowers clog vaporizers. Do not permit stems to enter your mix.

Stems found should be set aside. They can be chewed and swallowed for roughage. Seeds are uncommon in today's medical marijuana. If you find a seed, remove it.

4. When selecting a strain, squeeze it. If you can handle the medication, squeeze it for density. You want density. You want little fluff. Some strains look great, smell great, but once dry offer low yield and fluffy flowers. Stay away from airy flowers or whispy branches or long stemmed flowers. Think: density equals more flower. You want the strongest, most dense flower with the least amount of stem. Clubs package in their favor. That is, some clubs burn patients on medicine by loading it up with stemmed out flowers. Always buy flowers for these vaporizers, concentrates do not work. No medical hasish, resins, waxes, kief, or oil. Stay away from clubs who offer preground specials. Try to select a club with a clean, wide variety of strains priced no more than $40.00 for an eighth of an ounce. Shop around if prices seem high.

Clubs price top shelf strains for good reason but not all clubs price fair.

5. Find a club that offers delivery if you are recovering, in treatment, or if you don't want to drive with medication in your car. Clubs offer delivery. Find one. Most clubs will deliver anywhere you are including home, office, or your local coffee shop. San Francisco has several delivery clubs.

A Comparative Analysis of the Vapir bag inflatable, Magic Flight Launch Box, Arizer Solo, and Vapir NO2

Vaporizing is an art. It might appear to be effortless. It is not. It is a dance done with your breath and heat. It is learning to draw in at your most relaxed while pulling steady. Patients who are new to vaporizing will find the early attempts to be full of frustration. All four vaporizers make you wait for them to heat. They do not feature repeated inhalation. Each vaporizer has a refractory heating period after the patient draws from it. Unlike combustion based methods (like medical marijuana joints), vaporizers don't burn continuously. The closest approximation to repeated inhalation is using the Vapir bag inflatable with the optional whip in place of the bag. However, the singular bowl vaporizes quickly and is only feasible when patients are medicating together. The Vapir bag inflatable when fitted with the bag should be used in the following way: grind your medical marijuana flowers into a coarse powder, before turning it on, switch the fan on high (this is recommended in the manual), as soon as you turn it on, return the switch to low, set the temperature to 320 degrees. While it is heating, load the bowl and place the lid on it, place it in the drawer, slide the drawer in once the light turns green indicating Vapir has reached temperature, switch fan to high and inflate the bag. Once the bag is fully inflated, quickly detach the bag and cover with your finger to trap vapor. Turn device off. Inhale. If you want more volume in your vapor, increase the temperature to 325 degrees. Do not attempt to run medicine through more than once. The vapor produced on the second attempt is always harsh. If you are medicating with other patients, you can pass the bag, as it usually contains three to five full hits. You can also add another bag to the rotation. The bags tend to accumulate sticky residue from medicine. Bags may need to be gently pulled apart if the residue causes them to stick together which obstructs inflation. The Vapir bag inflatable does all the work. It is the only vaporizer with a fan. The Arizer Solo is the most user friendly amongst the three portables. To use the Arizer Solo: charge battery, turn unit on (and off) by pressing and holding both buttons, grind medicine to coarse powder (the Arizer can handle pieces of medical marijuana flower but ground flowers heat better), fill glass piece with medicine, place glass piece into unit once heated, allow unit to heat medicine until indicator light is on, draw. Once finished medicating, turn unit off by pressing and holding both buttons. Patients should keep Arizer Solo set to three. There are seven heating levels. Three is ideal for medicine. The Vapir NO2 should be set to 350 degrees. Hotter temperatures destroy flavor and lead to coughing fits. Some sensitive patients may try 345 degrees. Grind your medicine into a coarse powder. Fill the brass chamber to the top. Do not pack medicine in. You will hamper medicating. Allow NO2 to reach set temperature and draw steady. If you fail to get vapor, step away and wait. The moisture found in most strains will cause the temperature to drop during heating up. Once forty seconds have passed, draw again. The vapor should be robust, tasty, and visible. The NO2 will trick you into thinking all medicine has been vaporized. If you wait, you will get more vapor. If you are unsure about degree of extraction, inspect the medicine. Is it brown? If so, it has been vaporized. If it is still green or retains any smell, try it again. The expert's vaporizer is the Magic Flight Launch Box. This compact, heavy hitter is for the discrete patient. The device is made of Birch. It is a work of art. The batteries are rechargable and used to coax hits from this model of simplicity. The Magic Flight Launch Box features a cover that slides to reveal a trough made of mesh. Patients load the trough with coarse ground medicine before sliding the screen back over. The battery features a cap on the end for ease of applying pressure. Press the battery in and wait a few seconds. If you are using the mouthpiece, you will see an orange light followed by a vapor trail. Draw gently while firmly pressing the battery in. Count to seven. Shake the box. Exhale. You must shake the box as holding the battery for more than a few seconds causes combustion-like charring of the medicine and harsh vapor/smoke. The Magic Flight Launch Box batteries last the duration of one or two full troughs. Loading over the trough does not help with medicating. Excess medicine gets in the way and chars easily. The mouthpiece can be removed. Patients can draw directly from the hole for the mouthpiece. The Magic Flight Launch Box has the longest learning curve. The battery is sometimes difficult to gauge when drawing. That is, you don't know if you've got heat until you draw or if you wait too long you risk burning medicine. Once I mastered the four vaporizers, in terms of getting full extraction by using the above methods and settings, it occured to me to draft this comparison. It seemed unfair to each manufacturer to not medicate for several months with each device before publishing this analysis. All four produce the exact same post-vaporized browning of the flower, if used correctly with the above settings and methods. All four fully extract flavor, volume, and medicinal components of vapor. But, they have many differences in terms of method of heating, materials used for construction versus flavor retention, portability, durability, and for three of the four devices, battery life versus medicating needs. The Vapir bag inflatable was selected for price and easy comparison to market equivalents most patients cannot afford, namely the Volcano. The Vapir bag inflatable is a flagship vaporizer and represents the shift in technology from whip to bag. Early vaporizers featured a small piece of ceramic and a whip with a glass piece or a globe that collected vapor from a heating element positioned in the center. Patients would load the glass piece and place it on the heating element for the ceramic box vaporizers or draw from an attached tube for the globe vaporizer. The vapor was too harsh. Bag inflatables offered full extraction and a revolutionary smooth draw and exhale. The Vapir bag inflatable captures the essence of the technology and taste for an affordable price. Top shelf bag inflatables can run up to eight-hundred dollars. The Vapir bag inflatable retails for a little over a hundred. For patients

who are home bound, have difficulty
drawing or inhaling, or who want the
option to use a bag or whip, the Vapir
bag inflatable is ideal. It was the first
vaporizer to show up during my
treatment. It has incredible durability
and construction. It has consistently
delivered rich vapor. And, it is very user
friendly. Patients who are new to
medicating should consider the easy to
use Vapir bag inflatable. The main thing
to remember is to start with the fan
switch on high before immediately
switching it to low once powered on.
This directive is from the instructions
included with the Vapir bag inflatable.
From there, you set the temperature to
320 degrees. While the device is
heating, grind your flowers. Fill the bowl
and secure the lid. Insert the bowl into
the drawer. Insert the drawer once
device reaches temperature. Flip fan
switch to high and inflate the bag.
Remove the bag and inhale. Bags
include a cap. The instructions say bags
can be capped for up to an hour. I
suggest inhaling as soon as the bag is
full to get full flavor profiles. Letting
vapor sit makes it harsh or less flavorful.
Be sure to eject drawer and power down

after inflating. The bowl will be scorching hot. Do not touch it. I suggest flipping it over into a cooling dish of pyrex or clay. Most patients will have such a dish to hold all of the components for their vaporizer. Have an area to cool the bowl off. The Vapir bag inflatable comes with three bowls. If you are medicating with other patients, having preloaded bowls and extra bags is great. The other method of extraction is to use the optional whip. Patients go through the same procedure to medicate. The whip is attached in place of the shorter tube used to inflate bags. The vapor streams continously from the whip once you flip the fan switch to high. This is ideal for groups of patients medicating together. Advise others to not pull the whip to them. It can come out of the hole. The Vapir bag inflatable is made of high density plastic. It is the largest of the four devices compared. It can be hung by the strap for patients who want bags to inflate from above. I suggest using a stand of some kind. There is an optional table stand by Vapir but it positions the device straight up and down. After observing how the bags accumulate sticky residue from the vapors, my guess is the bags insides will stick worse than if the device is hung. The optional stand by Vapir starts with the deflated bag. The inside of the bag gets sticky which obstructs the inflation process. Hanging the device allows the bag to fill without the insides sticking to each other as much. And, if they do stick, the bag is easier to pry apart when inflating from a hanging position. Watch your fingernails when prying bags apart. Sharp or long nails can penetrate bags during pinching which can cause leakage. Five bags are included. They are durable but not indestructible. Be delicate with them and they will last. Another construction feature found in the Vapir is metal. The bowls used for medicating are metal and get hot. Patients medicating with other patients will invariably have a guest burn their fingers at some point. Be sure to warn others about the magnitude of heat from an ejected bowl. The Vapir bag inflatable is designed to deliver consistently rich vapor. The materials used detract some from the flavor but having a bag inflatable is worth it. For groups of patients medicating, the bag and whip can't be beat. The Vapir bag inflatable is not for patients who need compact size, discretion, and portability. If you are homebound, invest in one. It heats fast, produces a rich volume of vapor each time, and is fan powered for patients who have difficulty inhaling. The fan "inhales" for you into the bag. Patients will note residue accumulating on the insides of bags, once the bag sticks too much it can be placed in your recycling bin. The bowl accumulates the same sticky residue. The lid for the bowl can be gripped with needle nose pliers and caught on fire with a lighter to remove residue. The lid tends to get gummed up more than the bowl. The instructions suggest cleaning with Q-tips dipped in rubbing alcohol. This will work but if it does not, grip the metal and use a lighter to burn off the sticky residue. Pieces will become charred but it can be wiped off once cool. The tube from the device to the bag accumulates sticky residue. It can be cleaned with very hot water. The inside of the device builds up sticky residue. Most of which can be scraped from internal components. The Vapir bag inflatable bowl piece screens can wear down with use. Screens may detach and fray. Extra bags, cleaning utensils, bowls, and other replaceable pieces can be purchased from Vapir. The Vapir bag inflatable is an overall great purchase. The future designs should include the ability to set and keep the same temperature. Each time the device is powered off the user must manually reset the temperature. Other improvement might include a glass on glass optional whip and retractable legs for users who want the device to sit upright. The fan is audible. It can be disruptive for sensitive patients. A quieter fan may be included in future models. At the end of the day, patients who are using top shelf bag inflatables are still inhaling from a bag. Why pay almost a thousand dollars when there's a device that does an adequate job of producing the same result for a little over a hundred? Another reason to consider the Vapir bag inflatable is that vaporizer technology is moving away from bags and towards glass on glass for improved flavor extraction. The top shelf bag inflatable will become obsolete as technology moves towards maximizing volume of vapor and flavor extraction using glass components. Remember my oven analogy? If we are using convection, why not move into glass to improve vapor flavor? Medicine used is comparable to fine wine. If you are medicating, why not maximize flavor and enjoy the process? If you are faced with a difficult prognosis or terminal condition, medicine can include therapeutic effects, such as laughter. Medicine has been known to include euphoria. If that is criminal while you are facing uncertainty but it also helps you eat, so be it. Enjoy these devices. That brings me succinctly to the Vapir NO2 portable vaporizer. This is also a must have. Of all four devices, this one stands alone in that it can be plugged in or run from its battery straight out of the box. The packaging looks sharp and the device is more compact than the Vapir bag inflatable. It retails for closer to two hunded dollars. The NO2 opens up the world to the mobile patient. The device is made of high density plastic. It is too tall to fit in your pocket but can poke out without drawing too much attention provided the whip is detached and in another pocket. The whip should be put in a ziplock baggy when mobile. Going commando in your pocket invariably leads to lint sticking to the sticky residue inside the whip. If your whip is spotless, pocket lint will manage a way into the middle of it and you will inhale it when medicating. Using the NO2 at night requires a travel kit with a small flashlight. During the day, your kit should include: the bamboo stirring tool included in the box, a bag of preground flowers, a bag for post vaporized browned flowers (if you wish to retain for making butter and edibles), a lighter, any other item you use or need to maintain your NO2. Don't bother with the mouthpiece for the whip. You want the draw to be unrestricted. You can modify your NO2 by poking holes in the screens with a safety pin to increase airflow. Do not heat above 350 degrees. The NO2 screens must be cleaned regularly. The best method is to grasp them with needlenose pliers once extracted and burn off sticky residue with a lighter. The screens may appear charred but dust off once they cool down. The brass chamber for the medicine should never be hard packed. The screen lining the bottom of the chamber must be kept operational. Packing restricts your draw and wastes medicine. Fill it up. But, don't pack. The

NO2 set to 350 is ideal for patients who want a rich, flavorful vapor with full extraction. The NO2 makes the user wait but the reward is a dozen draws from one full chamber. When one considers the NO2 is made of plastic, uses a brass chamber, and a plastic whip, the flavor becomes surreal in quality. The NO2 is durable. It can take big drops. Scuffs may detract from its aesthetic appeal but have no impact on its function. The NO2 delivers. When it is plugged in and set to 350 the vapor stream is perhaps the most flavorful of all devices, including the Arizer. The design is logical but in the future could be pocket size for discretion and ease of transport. The battery life varies. If your medicine is moist more heating time will be needed to produce rich vapor at 350 degrees. This impacts battery life. Ambient temperature and wind impact battery life in that colder or more variable outdoor conditions cause the NO2 to work harder to reach 350 degrees. Battery life can last for two hours. If patients are sensitive and medicate with smaller amounts, battery life could last three hours. Extra NO2 batteries are available and can be charged and carried for long trips. Batteries are forty dollars each. The NO2 plugged in provides long medicating sessions. Users must wait in between draws for the chamber to reheat. But, the reward is full flavor extraction. The NO2 can function in groups of medicating patients provided everyone is aware of the reheating period required to produce quality vapor. The waiting period can be too long in large groups which is where your Vapir bag inflatable comes in handy. The NO2 is fickle with some strains and outdoor conditions when running from the battery. Vapor quality is somewhat compromised when running from the battery. Some cold outdoor conditions require the temperature to be raised by five degrees. The NO2 can frustrate patients new to vaporizing. The reheating period can be cumbersome for patients with small windows of time to medicate before their symptoms return. Future improvements could include a glass lined chamber and glass whip or optional fan for patients who have trouble inhaling. The size could become more compact and battery technology and life could be expanded.

The NO2 relies on screens, uses a brass chamber, and plastic. Yet, the flavor is retained. If you are looking for a tough, portable, durable, reliable vaporizer with good flavor extraction, grab the NO2. If cleaning, size, and limited battery life seem too much, consider the Arizer. The Arizer Solo portable vaporizer stands alone in this comparison in that it features a glass whip and ceramic heating element. It is half the size of the NO2 and fits easily in a pocket with the glass whip removed. It includes two glass whips and a potpourri dish. The battery outlasts the NO2. The Arizer is limited in that it only runs when off the charger. There is an adapter available that allows users to remain plugged in. But, out of the box, the Arizer is married to the charger. Once charged, the Arizer is powered on by holding both temperature buttons down for a second. The device beeps and lights up. Beeping can be turned on and off by holding the up button for a couple of seconds. The Arizer glass whip has one end for drawing and another for the medicine. Fill the end with coarse ground flowers. Set temperature to three. Allow the Arizer time to heat.

Remove the tab covering the heating chamber. Flip the Arizer upside down and place whip into it using both hands. If you try to place the whip right side up, you will spill medicine. Once whip is inserted, set right side up. Allow Arizer a solid minute to heat medicine, even if indicator light is on. Draw deep. Allow Arizer to reheat. Repeat as needed. The Arizer can also be positioned to seal over your glass waterpipe's stem. Remove your waterpipe's glass bowl. Set it aside. Coil a rubberband around the tip of the Arizer glass whip. This will function as a rubber seal. Allow the Arizer to heat but bump the temperature up to four. Place the glass whip with the rubberband over the stem and seal it by applying pressure. Draw from the waterpipe. Carefully set the Arizer down and allow it to reheat. Waterpipes can vary in size. Not all models will work. Visit your local retailer for a snug fitting waterpipe if you prefer medicating this way. Bring the (cleaned) glass whip with you to inspect the fit. Use ice cold water to cool the vapor if you are prone to coughing fits while medicating. When using the Arizer outside of your home, you need to include the following items:

a protective bag for the glass whip (velvet works or bubble wrap), the glass whip, the device, a toothpick, a bag of coarse preground flowers, a bag for browned flowers (if you are retaining for edibles and butter) and any other tool you use from home and a small flashlight for night use. The Arizer handles well in groups provided every one is told there is a waiting period between draws. The reheating period is brief in comparison to the NO2. The Arizer bounces back. When medicating in groups, patients should be coached on how to draw from the glass whip if using the waterpipe as an accessory. A proper seal means no air just vapor. Patients should be delicate with the glass whip. It is thick and well crafted but cannot withstand hard tapping out hence the toothpick. You need to gently stir and poke out browned flowers into your bag for them. Do not tap out the glass whip. Advise everyone not to tap the whip if the Arizer Is being used by a group of patients. They are nine dollars each. The only downside to the Arizer seems to be cleaning. The glass whip's shape makes cleaning a challenge with most implements. This is where my secret technique comes in handy. Go get a regular plastic drinking straw. Run hot water over and inside of the glass whip. Get it hot. Be very careful handling the glass whip as cleaning is the most likely time to break it. Take the drinking straw and begin ramming it into the drawing end of the glass whip. You must run hot water and vigorously scrub out the glass whip using the pointy edges of the crinkled plastic drinking straw. Steady hands are needed. The process takes as long as there is visible sticky residue. Keep poking the crinkled straw. If you need to, grab several straws and go to town on it. Be sure to keep a steady, solid grip on the glass whip. The interior chamber accumulates a sticky residue around the ring where the glass whip passes while being inserted. Invariably, some air and vapor escapes from the tiny space between the glass whip and chamber. This miniscule vapor air mixture slowly builds sticky residue which seems benign until you try inserting and removing the glass whip. It gets stuck. It causes the user to strain to insert and remove. The jerky corrective motion in the effort not to spill the bowl can lead to breaking the glass whip.

Clean the sticky residue from around the ring of the chamber at the point of insertion to avoid breaks. Glass itself can be considered a vulnerability and design weakness. I consider it a worthy sacrifice in the name of flavor. Be careful using the glass whip once its been fired. It gets hot. It can scorch skin. Resist the urge to test how hot it gets, you will injure your finger finding out. The battery life for the Arizer varies. If you are using it with small amounts, it can last up to five hours. Drop it from three to two once its heated if you want a thinner vapor but more battery life. If you are using the Arizer in conjunction with a glass waterpipe and setting it on four, your battery life will be shorter but not by much. Draws from the waterpipe are robust and seem to extract medicine faster from the flowers. This might account for the battery life difference. If you need to conserve battery power try this approach: turn Arizer on and set to three, take initial and follow up draws plus one more, turn down to two, draw twice, turn up to four, draw twice, power down. Future improvements might include: interchangable batteries, waterpipe adapted glass whip, a glass lined chamber, placement of charger plug on the side and ability to remain plugged in during use. The current placement of the charger plug is intentional. You are less likely to break the glass whip if you leave yours inserted between sessions if the device has to be on its side to accomodate the charger. Another factor for some patients is cost. The Arizer retails for up to three hundred dollars. I found mine for half that price. Shop around. The final vaporizer for comparison is the Magic Flight Launch Box or MFLB. This is the most compact vaporizer. It is also the only vaporizer made from Birch. The MFLB is for the traditionalist. It is classy and brings heavy hits to the table. The kit includes a travel tin, the device, two mouthpieces, the cleaning brush, two rubber bands to secure the lid in your pocket, two batteries, a velvet drawstring bag, two battery caps, a battery case, a charger, and an inscription engraved on the back to uplift and inspire. The MFLB is for seasoned vape enthusiasts. The patient starting out should know, practice makes perfect. You will need to be mindful of holding the battery in place too long.

Doing so creates combustion-like charring and smoke. The MFLB has to be felt out over time. Additional batteries can be purchased and there is an adapter for those who wish to be plugged in. The device offers unmatched portability. Load the trough. Close the lid. Place the rubber band on it to secure the lid. Grab the two charged batteries and off you go. The MFLB kit for longer outings should include the brush, a bag of preground flowers, a bag for browned flowers, one of the rubberbands, and fully charged batteries with one cap. The kit includes a velvet storage bag. Use it. Between full troughs, you will need to brush out the trough and mesh areas. Be sure to bring a small flashlight for night outings. Browned flowers get in crevices and must be brushed out. The taste from the MFLB is unique and flavorful. The Birch adds a layer of woodsy feel that will speak to the nature lovers. The MFLB is ultra discrete. Even with the battery inserted and mouthpiece, the MFLB is tiny. For patients who are sensitive to medicating and benefit from small doses, enjoy a more traditional feel to a vaporizer, and who want privacy and several large draws per battery the MFLB is a great buy. It retails for a hundred dollars. Get extra batteries. Batteries can power two or three full troughs. Small dosing patients will love stretching that out. The MFLB offers durability as well as a lifetime replacement policy. It won't shatter. It won't melt. Overall, the design is downright rugged. Patients introducing the MFLB to other patients will need to coach them at first. Start with the mouthpiece. The battery, once inserted, causes an orange light to become visible. A vapor trail begins to form and seep out. Allow just a moment for the battery to heat the medicine fully before drawing steady for several seconds then shaking the box to disperse heat and prevent charring. The perk to the MFLB is zero reheating time. You can rapid fire batteries until they are all tapped out. Take it camping. Other patients won't believe the draws until they achieve them with practice. The MFLB has carved its own path with its unique approach right down to the letter. They have cornered a unique market with their one of a kind device. This concludes the comparative analysis.

Buy all four vapes if you can. You can't go wrong. Enjoy.

BONUS SECTION: HOW TO GROW MEDICAL MARIJUANA

In researching the market for books on medical marijuana and vaporizers, I encountered many how to grow books. I felt obligated to add a section here for patients who have a prescription but cannot afford club prices or who just want their own medicine. Growing is going to be simplified for the sake of results not endless lecturing on the fine points. Medical Marijuana is a vigorous plant. It thrives in heat. For my method, you will be given a skeleton. It is up to you to flesh it out with details based on your living situation and local laws. You must acquire seeds or clones from your club. I will not provide suggestions on how to acquire illegal marijuana. Get clones or seeds from your local club. If you are not being prescribed medical marijuana, please do not use these methods. If you are ready to watch a life cycle through and become medicine in exactly one hundred fifty-nine days, get your green thumbs up! Growing is fun. Growing is science. Growing is art. Growing is sharing a bond with nature. Growing is educational and invigorating.

Growing can give you something
wonderful to distract yourself with if you
are homebound. You can sustain
yourself on a small investment in
equipment indefinitely. Growing offers
patients a joyful way to take part in their
own recovery by producing the very
medicine that will help them! Can any
other patient say that? Can you grow
Vicodin on a tree? No. Its manufactured.
And, to some degree, so is that beloved
club marijuana you spend hundreds of
dollars a year on. Growing bypasses the
club's price controlling. With your one
time investment for my method, you
control how much you need of what type
of strain. My method is not for large
scale growers. If you are hoping to learn
how to start a farm or your own
dispensary, I can't help you. I am going
to suggest some products by name. You
can buy there market equivalents but I
can't promise the results will be
comparable. To grow from seed, you
need to germinate seeds. If you are
using clones from your club, your
approach will change greatly. For either
situation, you need a light. My method is
for indoor growers. Growing outdoors
varies too much for this section. Look up

your region's planting season. In California, we harvest in the Fall. Find out when your planting season is and plant your germinated seed or clone. Water as needed. Let nature take over. It is that easy. Harvest and follow my directions for curing later in this section. Indoor growing allows you more control over environmental variables. If you are starting from seed, you will be proud of your medicine, like a parent. Clones are easy. We will reserve discussing clone selection and growing for later. To grow from seed, select seed stock based on attributes you find most helpful. Be sure to have some money set aside. Growing costs money. Plus, there's no guarantee your plants will make it. Growing can be challenging, frustrating, fruitless, and get expensive. My method aims to simplify the process for patients. You may want to grab a notepad for this section. You are going to need to take notes. You will have two areas for growing, a nursery and a budding area. To begin a crop from seed, you follow my instructions for germinating then you note the date your seedling sprouts first poked up and count ninety-nine days ahead on a calendar kept near the nursery on a wall next to a copy of your prescription. The 99th day you noted is the date they will go to the budding area for the last sixty days of their life. The nursery won't smell much. Therefore, it can be placed in more conspicuous places. The budding area will smell towards the end of the growing cycle. My method involves having a mini green house for seedlings with a heating pad that you water with a spray bottle. In the same area, you will have midrange size developing plants that are watered. As soon as you harvest, you place the midrange size developing plants to bud if they are ninety-nine days old or older. Remember, the life cycle is 159 days. You bud the last sixty days. You can clone your own plants before budding them and have an infinite cycle of harvests. Four or five plants produces plenty of medicine. Plus, you will have new finished batches every two months. The method will work without a hitch with daily care. The most pending question is where will you grow? The easiest way to solve that question is to get a fifty gallon aquarium. Stand it up. You will use this as your budding area, to finish your small crop of four or five plants. My method requires two lights. In the interest of keeping your costs down, I suggest using 150 Watt lights by Sun System. Why? They plug in to a regular wall outlet. They emit plenty of light to get exceptional results. They are cost effective in that they won't spike your power bill as high. Lights over 150 Watts might alert power company folks to activity. You will be running 300 Watts total. The other reason I use 150 Watt lights is to keep overall costs down. The heat produced by these lights is low compared to the lumens they emit. If you must, you can use a 250 Watt light in your budding area in the fifty gallon aquarium stood upright. But, for your nursery area, use the Sun System 150 Watt. Do not use flourescent lights for your nursery. Stem growth will be compromised. Heat from more powerful lights will cause this method to fail. Again, the maximum size for your budding area is 250 Watts. Anything over is too hot for the fifty gallon space.

You will need the following items to grow medical marijuana using my method:

1. Sun System 150 Watt Light x 2 (Optional 250 Watt Light for budding area)
2. Eight to ten gallon size plastic pots with a dozen drain dishes.
3. Super Sprouter Seedling Heating Pad & mini-Greenhouse. Mini-Greenhouse consists of two bottom trays and a see through plastic 6" or 7" propagation dome top that snaps into place over tray. The heating pad is placed in the bottom tray. The second tray is placed on top of the heating pad. The dome is snapped on top. Light penetrates from the dome and into the mini-Greenhouse which creates ideal seedling growth conditions due to the heat from the pad.
4. Grodan Stonewool AO-K Starter Plugs (get the one with 50 plugs).
5. Super Sprouter Seedling Heat Mat Thermostat.
6. Roots Organic Potting Soil (34 Lb. Bag).
7. Two timers.
8. Higromite (21.45 Liter Bags, buy two).
9. One Fiskars Softtouch Micro-tip Pruning Snip.

10. Three Spray Bottles.
11. Two watering cans.
12. Two small or medium size clamp-on fans.
13. Small bottle of Gravity Flower Hardener by Emerald Triangle.
14. Pura Vida Organics Grow (4 Liter).
15. Pura Vida Organics Bloom (4 Liter).
16. Olivia's Cloning Gel (2 oz.).
17. Two or three five gallon buckets.
18. A few lemons (to spike acidity in seedling water).

If you are starting from seed, take five Grodan starter plugs out. Fill a bowl with water and squeeze a lemon into the water. Dip the plugs into the solution. Remove and place on a on top of heating pad. Heating pad goes between bottom tray and top tray. Set thermostat on Super Sprouter Seedling Heat Mat Thermostat for germination. Place seed into hole in starter plug. Place the 150 Watt light no more than two feet above dome. Inspect plug for growth and moisture content after two or three days. Sprout should appear in a few days. As soon as the sprout appears count ninety nine days ahead on your calendar and note the date as this will be the day these seedlings will go to the budding area. If a plug loses moisture, fill a spray bottle with same lemon water solution and spray it down until moist. When you plug in the light, plug it in to the timer. You want the light to be on for eighteen hours a day and off for six. I suggest running it all day and timing it to go off at night. That way, if your nursery is in a lighted area, the added sunlight will only enhance growth. You want total darkness once the light turns off on the timer. No light of any kind can be in the nursery for the six hour dark period. The heating pad and clamp-on fan stay on twenty four hours a day. Do not plug them in to go off with the timer. For the first few weeks, you will spray the seedlings with the lemon water solution. You will marvel at their growth. Once they reach the top of the dome they are ready to be potted. Take enough Higromite to line the bottom of your gallon pot before filling the rest with Roots Organic Potting Soil. Dig a spot in the middle and place the plant, including the plug, and cover completely. On the same day you pot them, start four or five new seedlings. Remember, your first crop is unique in that you won't even turn the budding area light on until your plants are at least ninety-nine days old. You need to start a new batch of seedlings soon after potting the original plants. Once you pot those plants, start watering them with the Pura Vida Grow solution. Follow the instructions carefully. You mix a little Pura Vida Grow into water and the plants will thrive. Place them on the parameter of the dome under the light. Once you water them, return soon after and dump the runoff water from the draining dish underneath. If you leave it, bugs will thank you for giving them a place to reproduce and begin destroying crops. Just before you move the midrange size plants to bud, take some plugs and soak them in the lemon water solution. Read and follow the instructions for using the Olivia's Cloning Gel. You clip at a junction where there is branching. You dip the clipped end into the gel. You insert the gelled clipped end into the plug at a slight enough angle to prop it upright. Spray the leaves. Observe for several days. Rooting should occur. Soon, you will have a clone. It is ready to be potted and moved out to parameter once it touches the dome.

From now on, you simply clone before you move plants into the budding area. That way, you always have plants in the dome, outside the dome, and budding. The day you move your plants to the budding area is a joyous occasion. Find a way to hang the light inside the fifty gallon aquarium standing upright. Clamp your other fan on and aim it where the plants will be. The fan stays on twenty four hours a day. The light cycle changes once plants go to the budding area. Set the timer for twelve hours on and twelve off. Running lights during the day is more cost effective. Set your timer to go to total darkness at night. It is critical that no light enters the budding area during lights off. The aquarium is handy in the sense that you can cover most of it with foil to block out light. Leave the light, fan, and plant areas open. You can angle the aquarium as needed. Treat smell problems per space. Time release battery powered fragrance dispensers work well. Once plants enter budding area, begin using the Pura Vida Bloom to water them. Follow the instructions printed on the label. Be sure to note the date your plants were placed in the budding area.

Give them at least sixty days to bud.
You need to read the instructions for
using the Gravity Flower Hardener. It is
a miracle treatment that increases yield.
It must be applied in time to work.
Gravity will add yield if used correctly.
Using too much Gravity is
counterproductive. Make sure the plants
are not too close to the light source.
Leaves that turn brown or brittle at the
tops are withering from heat. Place your
hand palm down at the top of each
plant. If it is too hot for your hand, its too
hot for them. When watering, be sure to
empty drain dishes after waiting for
them to fill. Never leave standing water.
Bugs love it. Watching your first few
plants bud is sheer joy. Don't harvest
early, go by the calendar dates. Once
plants have matured and budded, clip
them using your snips. Hang each plant
upside down after trimming every single
fan leaf from it. You want it to be naked
except for the clusters of buds. Save
trim in paper grocery bags. Paper
grocery bags absorb moisture from the
trim. In two weeks, test squeeze a bud.
If it is dry, crisp, and crumbles, it is
ready. Buds should break off cleanly at
the stem. If they are sticky, moist, and

tough to rip off or leave a string, they
need to dry longer. Wait a week and try
again. Buds can then be stored in bags
or jars. Use Azamax if you encounter
bugs like aphids, billbugs, cucumber
beetles, cyclamen mites, earwigs,
fungus gnats, lacebugs, mealybugs,
rose chafers, sowbugs, spider mites,
spittlebugs, thrips, white flies and
nematodes. It takes care of other soil
borne critters, too. This list is not
exhaustive. Your goal is to produce
seedlings, then clones, with robust root
systems. Next, you pot them and place
them around the dome. After they
mature to ninety-nine days or older, you
place them in the budding area. You
harvest and move the next plants up.
The goal is perpetual harvest six times a
year of four or five plants. You must
keep all areas clean, ventilated, free of
bugs, and out of the light when lights are
off. You check on your plants daily.
Never go a day without checking them.
My method works because you spot
problems before they get bad if you
check your plants daily. Watering is
crucial. Do not over water. Follow
watering instructions on the Pura Vida
Grow and Bloom labels. Bugs and other

problems will show up on your plants. If you see problems, consult with local growers. Bugs are specific to your local climate. Azamax will prevail in most cases. Clones from your local club should be potted and placed in the budding area for sixty plus days. Clones from clubs are supposed to be female. Male plants are different in appearance from females. Clusters of empty seed pods are a tell-tale sign. Sometimes males go undetected until its too late. You will know when you squeeze a bud from a female plant you just harvested only to discover a multitude of seeds. Get an experienced grower to check your plant for gender if you are unsure. Seed stock from clubs claim to produce seedless female plants. That is why I have not spent too much time on how to differentiate plant gender. Growing your own medicine offers an unmatched role in your own healing process. You are able to witness the cycle of life then experience the plant's healing properties. If you have the means, try it. Growing is an affordable, rewarding, exciting, educational adventure. Nothing compares to loading up your new vaporizer with medicine you grew and

taking that first draw. Let medical
marijuana heal you. It will.

How to make Medical Marijuana Butter:

1. Get a crockpot. Turn heat to high. Put one pound (four sticks) of real butter inside crockpot. Allow butter to melt. Add water to keep butter from overheating. Once butter has melted, add four ounces of browned flowers from vaporizing or six ounces of trim from plants.
2. Stir the marijuana in and add enough water to float it. Turn heat to Low. Allow it to bond slowly over eight to ten hours. Stir the mixture and add water as needed. Too much heat vaporizes THC rendering your butter inert. Do not boil butter or heat above simmering.
3. After eight or ten hours of slow bonding, pour the solution through a screen to filter out leafy parts. Leftover leaf can be disposed of or put into brownie mix and cooked right away. The solution of water and butter should be poured into containers. Place the containers in the fridge.
4. The butter will float and separate from the water. Once the butter solidifies, poke around the edges

until the water can be poured out
from around the now solid butter.

5. Never use your medical marijuana
butter in the microwave. Never use a
microwave to melt medical marijuana
butter for use. Microwaves vaporize
THC. Try stirring spoonfuls of solid
butter into warm foods with dairy or
fat in them. THC bonds to lipids. Any
recipe or food that calls for butter
can be medicated. Enjoy!

This book is dedicated to Steve Jobs
who passed away the day it was
finished. Steve? I wrote every sentence
and my dissertation on Apple and iPad. I
filmed every game for my charity sport
on iPhone. I have a MacMini and a G5.
Thank you. Without your gifts, I couldn't
have a vehicle to share mine. Please
donate to Pancreatic Cancer research. It
took comedian Bill Hicks at a young
age, as well. Thanks for the good times,
Bill. We miss you.

www.ingramcontent.com/pod-product-compliance
Lightning Source LLC
Chambersburg PA
CBHW020438290526
45785CB00002B/903